Volume 3

The ART of Being Healthy

Real-Life Accounts of Children and Mothers Healing with Chiropractic

D0047992

DR. GILLES A. LaMARCHE, *Editor*

ISBN: 978-0-9898430-2-7

Library of Congress Control Number: 2016932640

Printed and bound in the United States of America

To hire Dr. LaMarche as a speaker at your next health and wellness event, you may communicate with him via email at drglamarche@gmail.com or on Facebook at Dr. Gilles LaMarche.

Cover & Text Design by Mary Jo Zazueta (tothepointsolutions.com)

Dedicated to all children who have suffered and to those who have found peace in their recovery. May you discover the life-affirming joy of optimum health and wellness.

A special thank you to Jeff Hays and Bobby Sheehan, producer and director of the critically acclaimed documentaries Doctored, Bought, *and* Undoctored *(www.jeffhaysfilms.com). We sincerely appreciate your commitment to exposing the truth in search of better health for humanity.*

CONTENTS

SECTION TWO: INFANTS
(Colic, Breast-feeding)

SECTION THREE: TODDLERS
(Bedwetting, Night Terrors)

SECTION FOUR: CHILDREN AND TEENS
(Migraines, Falls, Sports Injuries)

SECTION FIVE: IMMUNE SYSTEM
(Infections, Fevers, Failure to Thrive, Asthma)

SECTION SIX: BEHAVIORAL, NEUROLOGICAL, AND OTHER DIAGNOSES

The five most dangerous words in the English language:

Maybe it will go away.

Preface

Dr. Gilles A. LaMarche

The most precious gift in life is good health. If you don't believe me, ask anyone who is chronically ill or fighting a disease. Without hesitation, they will tell you that what they most want is "my health."

Likewise, if you ask any parent with a sick child what they would be willing to do to give their child good health, they are likely to say "Everything and anything."

The World Health Organization (WHO) describes *health* as follows: "Health is a state of complete physical, mental and social well-being and not merely the absence of disease or infirmity." This definition has not been altered since 1948; and yet, what we might call modern society has come to recognize health as being "the absence of symptoms and disease."[1]

Due to the quick-fix theory that so many live by, people think that the answer to all ailments can be found in the utilization of a drug or medication. Instead of focusing on the basis of good health, science has concentrated on trying to find the cause of disease and on defining the ability to fight disease.

What is today called *traditional medicine* works at eliminating or controlling signs and symptoms of a disease by utilizing chemicals and external invasive forces, such as surgery. It is mechanistic in nature, uses drugs to resist death, attempts to control the variables, and battles disease by attempting to take over the body's innate wisdom while working at relieving pain and postponing death. This is not health.

The *ART of Being Healthy: Real-life Accounts of Children and Mothers Healing with Chiropractic* is about bringing the

---

1. Preamble to the Constitution of the World Health Organization as adopted by the International Health Conference, New York, 19-22 June, 1946; signed on 22 July 1946 by the representatives of 61 States (Official Records of the World Health Organization, no. 2, p. 100) and entered into force on 7 April 1948.

truth to the surface and acknowledging that medicine, BIG Pharma, and the media can no longer expect to rule people with lies and deception.

The health care system in North America is in serious trouble. In both the United States and Canada, more money per capita is spent on health care than in other countries. We have become the product of commercialized propaganda and have made many decisions about health that actually lead to increased disease and morbidity. The U.S. makes up less than 5 percent of the world population, yet Americans consume more than 50 percent of prescribed drugs worldwide. (The use of over-the-counter and prescription drugs is not much better in my birth country of Canada.)

Many reputable and highly regarded researchers have provided information to governments that could serve to improve the health of our communities and save taxpayers billions of dollars; yet few of these ideas ever get implemented. Documentaries such as *Doctored*, *Bought*, *Undoctored*, and *Making a Killing: The Untold Story of Psychotropic Drugging* present facts that are hard to believe—and fatal to ignore.

The dedication of the majority of medical doctors is without doubt; the wonderful advancements that have taken place regarding crisis-care in medicine are obvious—and for that we are grateful. Yet, at the same time, there have been major abuses of power. The fact that pharmaceutical companies want to control everything that is perceived as health or health care is definitely a concern.

In the book *The Truth About Drug Companies*, it says: "Drug companies are involved in every detail of research, from design of the study through analysis of the data, to deciding whether to publish the results or not. That involvement has made bias not only possible but also extremely likely. Researchers don't control clinical trials anymore, sponsors do."[2]

According to the World Health Organization (WHO), the United States of America and Canada, which have great resources of scientific minds and technology, are not at the top of the healthiest countries in the world. As health care systems go, the WHO ranks Canada as having the thirtieth best health care system in the world, and positions the U.S. at thirty-seven.

---

2. Marcia Angell, MD. *The Truth About Drug Companies* (Random House, New York), 2005..

Under the heading "World's Healthiest Countries," Bloomberg rankings position the U.S. at thirty-three, Canada at fourteen, and Australia at third. To achieve better results with your and your family's health, you must be willing to think differently, to look at the available options, and to make wiser decisions.

Dr. Albert Einstein said:

"You cannot solve a problem with the same level of thinking that created the problem in the first place."

Therefore, we must encourage all politicians, taxpayers, and health care professionals to recognize the value shared in this book, and move toward a health care system that embraces and respects the human body's innate ability to heal.

Every spine might have a *subluxation* (displacement that affects the function of the nervous system). We know that each subluxation will lead to *dis*-ease, which in time could lead to disease. Potentially each subluxation needs to be adjusted, needs Chiropractic.

The developer of Chiropractic, Dr. B. J. Palmer said: "Every man, woman, and child has a spine. It makes no difference whether he or she is black or white, red or yellow, whether they live on a mountain or in a valley; on land or water; at the North Pole or the equator; rich or poor—it is equally applied."

It is our hope that these stories motivate you to research this exceptional healing art called *Chiropractic*, whether for your child, for another loved one, or for yourself.

Dr. B. J. Palmer also said:

"Potentially every sick person is demanding Chiropractic—calling for it, needing it, crying for it—actually shouting for it, but doesn't know."

"Many receive advice,
only the wise profit from it."

SYRUS

Introduction

Dr. Gilles A. LaMarche

I have the privilege of serving on the Executive Committee at Life University in Marietta, Georgia. The vision we embrace is:

Our goal is to maximize the expression of the perfection within.

We recognize that all organic systems in the universe are conscious, self-developing, self-maintaining, and self-healing.

We believe these systems work best when they are free of interference.

We understand that the nervous system is primarily responsible for orchestrating the internal and external dialogue of the body necessary for LIFE.

We acknowledge that there are three interferences to the nervous system: physical trauma, environmental toxins, and emotional stress.

Therefore, our purpose is to correct these interferences, allowing the organism to express its innate potential.

What you are about to discover inside this book are doctors who understand and practice this discipline; doctors who recognize that the human body is, in fact, self-developing, self-maintaining, and self-healing provided there is no interference; doctors who have the knowledge and ability to detect, analyze, and correct interferences to allow your body to heal.

Although some readers will consider each one of these stories a miracle, what chiropractors do is not miraculous. It is the application of true principles of healing that honor each human being's ability to heal. For more than three decades I have witnessed people healing when they were told that nothing could be done.

From this day forward, please recognize that physical and sometimes emotional symptoms are your body's signals that something is wrong. Don't let the pharmaceutical companies or others convince you to mask the problem by covering up the symptoms instead of addressing and fixing the problem. Be committed to getting to the root cause of what ails you and your children. Your life and that of your child depends on it.

This book will challenge some of your beliefs about health, health care, and healing. You might find yourself questioning what you have heard and learned from family, friends, physicians, and schoolteachers. As you read these stories, know they are firsthand accounts about ordinary people like you and your family who searched for the root causes of issues they were dealing with. Maybe it was excruciating pain during pregnancy, being told a C-section was necessary, an inability to breast-feed their newborn, colic, a diagnosis of "failure to thrive," severe asthma, repeated ear infections, anxiety, etc. Regardless of the issue, once interference was removed through Chiropractic care, the body (and even the mind) healed.

While selecting the stories to include in this book, I often cried tears of sadness for what the children and parents had to endure; then tears of joy would well up and make reading nearly impossible when I realized their persistence to choose a different path that led to healing. I think you are about to experience similar emotions.

About the Editor

DR. GILLES LAMARCHE was born and raised in Timmins, Ontario, Canada. A Bachelor of Science graduate of the University of Toronto (1975), he later earned a Doctor of Chiropractic degree from Toronto's Canadian Memorial Chiropractic College in 1979.

After twenty-five years of active practice, Dr. LaMarche decided to share his passion and talents at Parker University in Dallas and with Parker Seminar attendees around the globe, from 2006 to 2012. In 2013, he joined the Executive team at LIFE University in Marietta, Georgia. His unequivocal passion to share health information to empower people to make informed health care choices for themselves and their families has led him to write numerous books and articles, and to share his knowledge and wisdom with audiences around the world.

The Art of Being Healthy is part of his communication strategy to allow multiple chiropractors to share their wisdom and experiences with an international audience.

For more information or to book Dr. LaMarche as a speaker, you may communicate with him via email at **drglamarche@gmail.com** or on Facebook at **Dr. Gilles LaMarche.**

To all the children of the world
who are born wise and pure,

To their parents who seek wisdom
in making proper choices,

To all healers who seek to
help human beings thrive,

To all teachers who persevere,

To all mentors who help raise the bar,

To all patients who give healers
enlightenment and courage to continue,

And to you, our readers, for your willingness
to learn and make better choices.

Cherish the past,
embrace the future,
and celebrate life to the fullest
through Chiropractic.

SECTION ONE

Pregnancy and Delivery

Our goal is to bring forth knowledge
and information that will guide you
to experience increased
health and well-being.

From Against to Advocate

Dr. Claudia Anrig

Twelve years ago, when I was pregnant with my daughter, I didn't know anything about prenatal Chiropractic care. I also didn't know that a car accident I had been in eight years before she was conceived could affect her delivery.

When I checked into the hospital three weeks before my due date to have labor induced, I expected my delivery to be perfectly normal and that everything would be fine. I was wrong.

Twenty-seven hours after labor was induced, and after four hours of pushing labor had no results, my midwife consulted with an obstetrician. He determined that Mikaela was stuck in the birth canal. My pushing wasn't moving her any closer to delivery, and her heart rate was decelerating to a dangerous level. The obstetrician asked my husband and me if he could use a vacuum extractor—although we really didn't have a choice because he said they were losing Mikaela.

The doctors attached the suction cap to my baby's head and began pulling as I pushed. When her head cleared, I remember a short-lived sense of relief, until the doctor informed us that Mikaela was wedged tight. Apparently, one of my hips hadn't spread properly—undoubtedly due to the earlier car accident, and there wasn't enough room for her shoulders to get through. The doctor informed my husband, Michael, and me that he was doing everything he could, but he was losing both of us. Then he reached in and wrenched Mikaela out.

The rest is just a blurry nightmare. I went toxic at the moment of delivery, and Mikaela looked dead. I watched from across the room as two hospital personnel each held one of my baby's ankles and flicked the bottom of her feet trying to get

1

her to cry. Mikaela never made a sound. They rushed her from the room to the NICU.

I refused treatment for the toxemia until someone told me what was going on with my baby. I remember lying in shock as a pediatrician I didn't know gave me a sterile list of the problems facing my newborn. Her Apgar scores were 4 and 6; she was fighting for her life; she was on IVs and oxygen; and her left arm was completely numb. I asked the doctor if her arm was going to atrophy. He informed me that was *the least* of Mikaela's problems; but, yes, it could. He said something along the lines of, "*If* she makes it, she'll need a couple of surgeries, and then she *might* regain *some* feeling in her arm."

This doctor was not Mikaela's pediatrician. Dr. Judi Krogstad was on vacation the night Mikaela was born, and he was one of her colleagues. I had researched pediatricians, and Dr. Krogstad was the best in the county; this guy, not so much.

We spent the next six days in the hospital recovering. Upon her return, Dr. Krogstad saw Mikaela every day. My baby was slowly improving, but we still had several frightening moments. The first time Mikaela was brought to me, she was three days old; and two hours later, her body temperature dropped to a dangerous level. I didn't even get to keep her with me in the hospital room until she was five days old.

I was also having breast-feeding issues, but Dr. Krogstad was certain we just needed to get home and everything would work itself out.

The day we were released, Dr. Krogstad informed me that Mikaela was still in some danger and that she wanted to see her every day at 2:00 p.m. for the next week—including Sunday.

The next day, I took Mikaela to her appointment. Dr. Krogstad was pleased to hear that she had started breast-feeding as soon as we were home. The doctor was still concerned about the baby's color and ordered another bilirubin test. While this was being done, she informed me that Mikaela had a brachial plexus injury—damage to the network of nerves that sends signals from the spine to the shoulder, arm, and hand.

She wanted me to make an appointment for Mikaela to be seen by Dr. Claudia Anrig. I assumed Dr. Anrig was a pediatric orthopedist or a neurologist. Dr. Krogstad said, "No, she's a chiropractor."

Well, I'm sure I looked at her like she had just sprouted a second head out of her neck. That was *insane*! I told her I'd have to talk with my husband about it; I was sure he'd think the concept was as crazy as I did.

My only experience with Chiropractic had been after my aforementioned auto accident. That man was not a good chiropractor, so I had pretty much written off the whole profession.

When we returned home that day and my husband called to see how Mikaela's appointment went, I told Michael about Dr. Krogstad's referral. He told me to see if Dr. Anrig was a provider on our insurance—like he was actually entertaining the idea. I was appalled.

The next day, Dr. Krogstad asked me if I had called Dr. Claudia yet. I stalled. I told her I had to see if she was a provider on our insurance. She was.

The next day—and in the days following—I continued to stall. On the seventh day, when Mikaela was just thirteen days old, I took her to her final appointment. Dr. Krogstad took one look at Mikaela and said, *"This baby has not seen Dr. Claudia!"*

I remember looking down, feeling a little ashamed of myself, but also concerned that I had run out of excuses. When I looked back up, Dr. Krogstad was staring at me with steel in her eyes and said, "I have given you *sound medical advice*, and you're not taking it. Either you call Dr. Claudia Anrig *today* to make an appointment for this baby, or I'm going to report you." She was loud and vehement; and I stood there in shock.

Dr. Krogstad stomped out of the room. I dressed Mikaela and left. I cried all the way home, warring with my own fears. I was still crying when my husband called at his usual time to check on the baby. He asked what was wrong with her, and I said, "Nothing." So he asked why I was crying. "Dr. Krogstad *threatened* me!" I said.

I remember Michael asking why we had picked Dr. Krogstad. I told him she was the best pediatrician in the county. He said, "Well, if the best pediatrician in the county is this adamant about it, what's the problem?" Isn't it just like a man, to cut through all the emotional nonsense and get to the root of the matter? So, I hung up and called Dr. Claudia's office.

Over the next seven months, Dr. Claudia helped us through constipation, ear infections, colic, and a horrible bout with thrush. Then, one day, when Mikaela raised both arms over her head for the first time, I cried! In that emotion-filled moment, I had *no idea* that this symbolic gesture would take on a life of its own, touching hearts and minds well into my baby girl's future.

It was just a few short months later when I made the mistake a lot of mothers make: I dropped out of Chiropractic care. Mikaela was all better—right? *Wrong!*

By the time Mikaela was three, she was suffering from allergies so bad she'd wake up gagging and vomiting from post-nasal drip. Mikaela was four when she started seeing Dr. Claudia again. Within a few years, no more allergies, no more annual colds, no more chronic ear infections ... no more problems. Period!

But that's not where the story ends. I now work for Dr. Claudia, helping her help other Family Wellness Chiropractors have the same kind of relationship with their local pediatricians like the one she had with Dr. Krogstad. Through Dr. Claudia's mentoring program, I help her help other chiropractors educate their patients on the benefits of Chiropractic care for children. I travel around the country with her; and when I come home, the first question my daughter asks at the airport is *not*: "What did you bring me?" It is: "How many times did you tell my story, Mom?"

Mikaela knows how important her story is; she understands that more parents need to know this truth. The simple fact is: my ignorance could have cost my daughter the use of her left arm. Today, everywhere that Dr. Claudia and I are privileged to speak, Mikaela's story is touching hearts and minds.

And me? I've changed from being against Chiropractic to an advocate!

Anastasia Line, Parent & Chiropractic Advocate
and Business Administrator
Dr. Claudia Anrig's Family Wellness Education
Fresno, California
www.drclaudiaanrig.com

Summer in the Summer

Dr. Tracy Wilson

It was early July and we were excited for the arrival of our daughter. The room was painted, all quilts and blankets were cleaned and fluffed. We anticipated an amazing celebration as we welcomed our new family member into our apartment. The day started out normal for me, up early and off to school. My wife shuffled down the stairs and made the drive to work. In the middle of her shift, her water broke.

She messaged me on my pager, but used the old "code" for "this is about to happen"; so I ignored the message—but it kept coming. I finally called to hear: "Dallas Medical City, how may I help you?"

Shivers went through my spine. We were about to start a test at Parker College of Chiropractic and now I was fleeing the school to get to my daughter's birth. I made it in time, but barely.

Within an hour of my arrival, Summer, joined the world! She was gorgeous and perfect. We cuddled her in the following moments and dealt with emotions that only a child can bring.

A few minutes later, the doctors took her from us to start the weighing and measuring process; and then the unthinkable happened, she stopped breathing. They rushed Summer out of the room and down to ICU. We followed in shock. Through the small window, we watched, cried, and prayed for our daughter. From complete joy to complete brokenness, we stood clueless, as to what the next moments would bring.

For nine days we sat in ICU while they tested, poked, probed, and monitored her. The doctor finally told us, "We do not know why these things happen; we just have to give her some drugs and monitor her."

We asked, "Why the drugs? What are they for? How do we know they are right?"

In answer, all he said was, "We don't know. This is just what we do."

My heart sank. I knew God made the body to function and not to fail. I knew there was more, but I was stuck, confused, and broken.

As I walked through the halls at Parker College, I came across a professor of mine, Dr. Michael Hall. I asked him if anything in the spine could make this "Sleep Apnea" process change. He rattled off a whole bunch of neurology that I had no clue about. I recorded it, and memorized it. Then, I asked the Pediatric ICU doctor about it. I recited what Dr. Hall had said, only by memory, and prayed the doctor didn't ask me any questions.

The PICU doctor said, "That is how it is supposed to function, but for some reason, in these cases, it doesn't." He patted me on the back and walked off.

I cried, and thanked God for showing me a way. We checked Summer out of ICU and took her to a Pediatric Chiropractor who adjusted her atlas. The monitor normalized right in front of us.

Today, Summer is twenty years old, beautiful, and full of life. She has finished her third year at university. On a daily basis, I wonder what life would have been if I had not known about Chiropractic and if she had not been adjusted from birth to now. I thank God for giving us this powerful example of how Chiropractic saves lives.

This knowledge and understanding has driven me to teach Chiropractic around the world and to have a practice that is focused on children. Our practice is fifty percent kids and full of families. We have had dozens of "Summers" in our practice—children who have discovered vibrant health because of Chiropractic.

I hope you choose Chiropractic for life and for the life of it.

Tracy Wilson, DC
8004 Abbeville
Lubbock, TX 79424
www.CreateYourWellness.com

Pregnancy Should Not be Painful

Dr. Amanda F. Jerviss

I first met Jennifer at a natural parenting expo. One of my patients who had gone to college with Jennifer, saw her in the parking lot and sent her to my booth. Even though Jennifer was in her mid-twenties, she looked worn-out and tired. She was with her husband and their two-year-old son.

We talked briefly about how the nervous system controls all functions of the body and Jennifer told me that she'd had some complications when her son was born. She made an appointment to come to my office for an exam. When she told me her story, I was blown away.

When her son was born at a birthing center, she pushed before she was completely effaced. The midwife held her cervix open and she had internal tearing that was more extensive than the midwives were prepared to suture. She was transferred to a hospital, where she was painfully sutured without anesthesia. She was traumatized both physically and emotionally by the experience, and diagnosed with post-traumatic stress disorder.

Two years later, Jennifer was still in constant pain. She had been to several medical doctors and was taking several strong medications. Some of the medications were causing her violent dreams and hallucinations. Unfortunately, she had no resolution. She could not stand for more than five minutes without intense, burning pain in her vaginal and pelvic floor areas. Wearing any type of pants, even pajamas, resulted in extreme pain in her groin area. She was now beginning to lose hope that she would ever improve.

After taking X-rays and examining her spine, I adjusted her sacrum and second cervical vertebra. She immediately felt some relief. She came in twice per week for several weeks; and each time I saw Jennifer, she had noticeable improvement in her health.

Prior to coming to my office, she had accepted an invitation to be an attendant at a friend's wedding. Jennifer feared that she would need to sit at the front of the church during the wedding ceremony because standing was too painful. After a few weeks under my care, the wedding day arrived. When she came back from the wedding, she excitedly reported that she was able to stand during the entire ceremony with minimal pain! Her life was improving!

I began adjusting Jennifer at the beginning of May, and by August, she was not only able to wear loose-fitting pants, she was able to wear jeans. Today, she can play with her son. She is free to be the person she wants to be, and she rejoices that she can do activities with her family that she thought she had lost forever. Her entire appearance has changed from when I first met her—Jennifer is vibrant again.

I am grateful to have played a part in her healing, and I am grateful that her friend told her about Chiropractic and my practice. Jennifer is now expecting her second child and has continued to be adjusted regularly over the past two and a half years. She recently told me that this pregnancy has been remarkably better than the first one. She has less low-back and sciatic pain, a condition that she previously thought was an unavoidable part of pregnancy.

> God made the human body to function wonderfully, and to heal. Chiropractic unleashes that ability!

Amanda F. Jerviss, DC
Jerviss Family Chiropractic
www.VibrantSpine.com

Mrs. Hill and Baby Garrett

Dr. Chelsea Pearson

Mrs. Hill came to the office when she was twenty-one weeks pregnant with her third child. She complained of low-back pain, left-hip pain, and numbness in her left leg with weight bearing. She explained that with each pregnancy, she had left leg/hip pain and premature labor, to the point of requiring bed rest.

At twenty-eight weeks, they found the baby engaged and breech in her pelvis. She was put on bed rest for premature labor and given meds every four hours to stop labor from developing. Throughout the eight weeks of bed rest, her low-back pain progressed significantly. She also developed upper-back and neck pain, headaches, and blood clots in her legs. She was then administered blood thinners, at two injections a day to slow down the clotting.

At thirty-six weeks, she was pulled off bed rest. After four adjustments, including the Webster technique, Mrs. Hill went into labor on her own and the baby was born at thirty-eight weeks, head down, with no complications.

However, two weeks after his birth, Garrett started to have difficulty latching onto his mom's breast, especially the left. He became super fussy, tense, increased gas, was not comfortable on his back, and had projectile vomiting followed by a painful cry. After one week, the projectile vomiting was progressively worse, to the point that it would happen after every feed. In addition, it was followed by a painful cry.

After doing some research, Mrs. Hill realized she had two options: stop nursing and use formula with medication, or nurse and see a chiropractor. When Mrs. Hill brought Garrett into the office, he was tense and rigid. He favored his left side and curved his body to the left. His head was right rotated with a left-head tilt. He also had a tight jaw and difficulty opening his mouth.

After one adjustment, his reflux significantly decreased. After four adjustments, his reflux was 90 percent improved. Garrett's mom reported that he no longer cries after his feedings; she is able to nurse him 100 percent, with no supplementing; he is gaining weight; he is able to turn his head; he nurses on both sides; and presents as the happiest baby.

Chelsea Pearson, DC, FICPA
Thrive Chiropractic
1230 N. Northwood Center Court, Suite A
Coeur d'Alene, Idaho 83814
208-665-9688
www.thrivecda.com

Amy's Story

Dr. Claudia Anrig

When Amy arrived at my office, she was thirty-six weeks pregnant and upset that she was going to need a C-section because her baby was breech. She had heard that the Webster Technique might help and was hoping it was true.

Dr. Larry Webster, a chiropractor, developed a Chiropractic technique that can be utilized on women during their third trimester. This special technique evaluates the position of the sacrum (tailbone) to see if it is in the correct or incorrect position; provides a gentle adjustment; and, with a light thumb contact on the belly, relaxes the ligaments and muscles anteriorly (in front) to produce faster results.

I told Amy she was in the right place because, not only could I do the Webster Technique, I was one of only two instructors Dr. Webster had approved to teach his work. The Breech Mal-position technique is one that I developed (Webster Advance-developed by Anrig) and showed Dr. Webster how to perform on his patients.

I explained to Amy that the technique was not an obstetrical procedure and assured her it was very safe and most effective the earlier we got started.

I also informed her that a breech presentation was common with first-time pregnant moms (which she was) and that her tight abdominal muscles and ligaments may cause something called "In-Utero Constraint."

In-Utero Constraint can happen not only in breech positioning, but also transverse, face/brow or oblique lie in the last trimester. The best position that babies innately move into (or naturally should move into) is the vertex or head down position during the seventh month.

With a fetus in the wrong position in the last trimester, it is not uncommon for them to develop any of the following: torticollis, lactation issues (neck or jaw out of alignment), reflux, colic, discomfort in any position, constipation, and difficulty sleeping. The infant may also develop immune issues, be slow on their milestones, or have behavioral issues as they become older. So, I also encouraged Amy to have her little one checked after he was born.

With just four visits, the baby safely turned (to the surprise of her OB—with whom she promptly shared her Chiropractic story and the Webster Technique). After that, we checked Amy weekly until her due date. This was the best for her because Amy had never had Chiropractic care growing up and, as a gymnast and cheerleader, she had many spills and falls with impact directly to her tailbone. We wanted her sacrum to stay stabilized.

Ethan was born quickly (something pre-natal chiropractors hear all the time from their patients) and two days, later she brought him in for his checkup. Her lactation specialist had also told her that his right jaw was not opening correctly and that she might want to see a chiropractor.

With a very gentle exam of touching and palpating Ethan's neck and jaw, it was discovered that his atlas (top vertebra in the neck) was slightly out of alignment and he potentially had temporomandibular joint disorder (TMJ) on the right. Ethan had his first adjustment and responded immediately by latching on strongly and breast-feeding without any further issues.

Both Amy and Ethan are currently enjoying Wellness Chiropractic Care, which may be new for some who believe that you should only see chiropractors when you are hurting. When Amy and her husband were thinking about having a second child, we started them both in Pre-Conception Chiropractic Care—evaluating nutrition, exercise, and stress-relief before conceiving.

Claudia Anrig, DC
www.drclaudiaanrig.com

The Quest for VBAC

Dr. Katherine A. Kadin

After a traumatic birth experience that led to a C-section, Kimberlea was determined to have an unmedicated vaginal delivery with her second baby. When we met a couple years ago, despite receiving regular Chiropractic care, she was suffering from extreme left hip and back pain, to the point where she could barely lift her left leg.

She asked her chiropractor why she was in so much pain, and no answers were forthcoming. His specialty, though fantastic, was geared to athletes. This left Kimberlea seeking to receive Chiropractic care from someone specifically trained in pregnancy and the Webster Technique, a specific sacral adjustment designed for pregnant women. Her doula and nutritionist suggested a consult with me, since I am specifically trained in the Webster Technique.

Kimberlea procrastinated contacting me for a while because she didn't want to "cheat" on her chiropractor, but at thirty-two weeks she was told that her baby was breech. She left the sonogram saddened by the news because her chances of having a VBAC (vaginal birth after cesarean) were being dashed because of her baby's position.

She immediately called my office and took the first available appointment. After the first adjustment, Kimberlea felt better. She could lift her left leg, and had hope that the baby would have a chance to turn. She began to see me once or twice per week, as often as she could manage. She hoped to improve her pain relief and increase the odds of the baby turning due to the optimized pelvic alignment. After receiving adjustments, she was able to sleep better at night. The adjustments also released tension that had built up and her baby went vertex (head down).

The Webster Technique helped create the alignment and space necessary for Kimberlea's daughter to turn head down. Kimberlea knows Chiropractic is the main reason she succeeded; so I now have the pleasure to be caring for her during her third pregnancy.

Katherine A. Kadin, DC, DACCP
Kadin Family Chiropractic & Wellness Center, LLC
6212 Montrose Road
Rockville, MD 20852
240-430-1004
www.KadinFamilyChiro.com

What Pregnancy Should be Like

Dr. Katie Greeley

In my many years of being a chiropractor, I have been honored to care for many pregnant women. There are so many changes that happen with pregnancy. Each trimester offers its challenges; often in different ways. To be a part of that new growth and care for expectant mothers is astounding. I have many encouraging stories. I have chosen to share a few that most inspired me.

A woman newly pregnant with her third child came to my office because people told her Chiropractic could reduce her back pain and ease her labor. While taking the history of her first two pregnancies, I learned that she labored for forty-two hours delivering her first child and thirty-eight hours for the second. She had sciatica with both previous pregnancies and was looking to have a better pregnancy with the third baby. She was making a wise choice by seeking assistance during her first trimester. Throughout her care, we explained how the joints of her spine and pelvis work. This led her to understand that when the pelvic joints are well aligned and balanced, allowing for natural movement of the pelvis, the likelihood of the sciatic nerve being impinged goes down tremendously.

During this pregnancy, she experienced minimal low-back and occasional, yet slight, sciatic pain. She followed through with her Chiropractic care, and even stopped in for an adjustment on her way to the hospital. She delivered in less than eighteen hours, half of her previous labor time. She was thrilled.

Another case is a woman who was pregnant with twins, a boy and a girl. We started seeing her at the beginning of her second trimester. She wanted a natural birth but the babies were in the yin/yang position. The boy was head down and the girl was frank breech.

Her current OB/GYN would not deliver a breech baby because he had not done so in the last twenty years. He also told her she would be lucky to make it to thirty-five weeks. Well, that little girl must have flipped around at least eight times during the course of our treatment. One day she would be breech; then after an adjustment, she would be head down. The mother had convinced the OB/GYN to allow her to deliver the first baby vaginally and then ultrasound in between to see if the girl did, in fact, follow her brother and stay head down. So, at thirty-eight weeks, when the mom's water broke and she went into labor, her daughter stayed head down and she was able to deliver both babies naturally.

Another case is about letting moms know their due dates. Not everyone has a forty-week gestational period; so when a client chose to listen to her body, she was able to deliver a healthy baby at forty-two weeks without extra help, such as an epidural or other interventions.

We always encourage women to listen to their bodies. With Chiropractic keeping the pelvis in alignment and the spine free of subluxations, women get the chance to enjoy their pregnancies as a natural life occurrence, with little to no symptoms.

The body works miracles every day. To help minimize the symptoms of heartburn, swelling, low-back pain, and headaches by removing interferences along the spine, we chiropractors are facilitators of health and wellness. We allow the women in our practices to enjoy the experience of being pregnant rather than dreading it. We are also one of the few places where women can lay face down on our pregnancy pillows in their second and third trimesters.

Katie Greeley DC, CACCP
Certified in Family Wellness, including Prenatal and Pediatric Care
10815-3C FM 2222, Ste. 100
Austin, TX 78730
512-234-1868
www.austinwellnesschiropractic.com

Infertility to Pregnancy

Dr. Kimberly Harper

Being a doctor of Chiropractic, we often take the miracles we see in practice for granted. I was reminded of that lesson with one of my employees, Corey. Corey was a new addition to my team and had never experienced Chiropractic care before. Like most of the employees who work with us, she heard stories from patients of the great results they were getting with Chiropractic and asked if she could be a patient as well. I always love taking care of my staff because I hope for them to be as healthy as possible; not only so they can feel fantastic, but also have abundant energy and excitement to share with the patients that come to us for help.

During her consultation, Corey shared that she had been involved in a serious car accident six years ago and had many low-back and pelvic issues ever since, making her stiff and sore. Even mild exercise was difficult.

We started working with Corey's spine and nervous system, and gradually she noticed her range of motion increasing and her pain levels consistently decreasing. She even started exercising more consistently.

A couple of months into her care, she asked if having misalignment in the low back and pelvis could cause any female issues. I explained to her that the nerves that control the female organs do come from that area of the spine, and if there is nerve interference caused by misalignment, it could decrease the ability of the organs to function correctly. Obviously, the better nerve flow a tissue or organ receives, the better it will function.

Corey then shared that she had been married for four years and they had been trying to get pregnant since their wedding, with no results. She and her husband looked into infertility treatment and adoption because they just were unable to conceive. I told Corey that we would continue to work with removing the nerve interference and see what happened.

A couple more months went by, we continued adjusting Corey, and she continued to improve. One morning I came into work to find a card on my desk and an anxious Corey waiting outside my private office door. I opened the card and read her fantastic news: Corey was pregnant! We were both so excited that I started to cry tears of joy. I continued to care for Corey through her entire pregnancy and she delivered a healthy baby boy. Corey decided to be a stay-at-home mom after her baby was born; and ironically, the woman I hired to replace her got pregnant the next month too!

Kimberly Harper, DC
Family Care Chiropractic
Fishers, IN 46038
www.familycarechiro.net

From Infertility to Childbirth

Dr. Laura T. Brayton

As a chiropractor specializing in maternity and pediatrics, I have seen multiple families positively touched through the power of Chiropractic care. However, one story in particular will stay with me for the rest of my life.

Last summer, I gave a lecture on preconception health that J and her husband attended, as they were excited and anxious to start a family soon. The anxiety revolved around J's diagnosis of PCOS (polycystic ovarian syndrome), a common hormone disorder, at the age of seventeen. Her gynecologist had told her it would be difficult for her to get pregnant and sustain a healthy pregnancy.

After hearing my talk, J began Chiropractic care with the hope of improving her fertility. In addition, lifestyle modifications were established, many she researched on her own as she was fully committed to living a healthy lifestyle. She conceived a few months later on the first attempt, a far cry from what she had been told at seventeen.

I had the honor of supporting J's ever-changing body throughout the pregnancy. I also empowered her to create the birth of her dreams: an unmedicated vaginal delivery.

J is a testament to the power of living a fully conscious lifestyle through education and commitment to evolve beyond the limitations often put on us by others.

One year after starting regular Chiropractic care, J gave birth to a healthy baby boy. She chose to name her son after me, Brayden. This is the highest compliment I have ever received and I am so grateful that I had the opportunity to serve this family.

I truly believe that the body is completely capable of self-healing at every level and I love to inspire those around me to experience transformation.

Laura T. Brayton, DC, CACCP
Hoboken Chiropractic + Wellness, Inc.
50 Harrison St., Suite 316
Hoboken, NJ 07030
201-792-3544
www.HobokenChiro.com

The Value of Gonstead Care

Dr. Laura Stone

The following testimony of Anna and her family will allow you to see the difference Gonstead Chiropractic care had on her body during two very different pregnancies, labor and deliveries; and how continual care for her family has added to their wellness lifestyle.

Adult care: Anna had a bout of low-back pain when her first child, Olive, was almost one year old. After graduating to maintenance care, Anna started taking advantage of the health benefits that Chiropractic care adds for one's body. She states, "Pain relief being one, but I also noticed an increase in energy and an improvement in skin clarity as a healthy side effect."

Prenatal care: Anna continued to be adjusted monthly throughout her second pregnancy and was blessed to deliver a happy and healthy baby girl named Sadie. She contributes that success to regular maintenance care throughout her pregnancy and has not experienced the same hip, low back and knee discomfort that she experienced after Olive was born.

Delivery: Anna states, "My labor with Olive was nearly twenty-four hours. I had Pitocin for half of that time; with an epidural for seven hours for pain relief. I had to push for an hour and a half and, even with intervention, I was unable to push very effectively. My second baby, Sadie, was similar, needing few medical interventions; however, the length of labor was cut drastically. Pitocin was needed for only two hours and the epidural for twenty minutes (which wasn't enough time, since I was fully dilated much sooner). Less than ten minutes of pushing and she was welcomed into my loving arms." Anna adds,

"I know without a doubt that my well-adjusted body was able to adapt better to a growing baby during pregnancy and much more equipped to handle a delivery the second time around."

Postpartum: Anna states, "My healing and recovery time was significantly faster and easier after Sadie. I had little to no low-back and hip pain after delivery and upon returning home with child. Compared to my first delivery, which brought much swelling and fluid retention throughout my body, the later delivery I noticed my fluids regulating much faster with minimal swelling. I just felt healthier!"

Infant adjusting: Sadie's first Chiropractic adjustment was when she was three weeks young. This critical adjustment allowed us to locate any nerve interference resulting from intra-uterine constraint and the manual force used during delivery. Sadie continues to do well with breast-feeding, bowel movements, and her body has been able to adapt more effectively as increased immune function is evident during environmental stress.

Toddler adjusting: When Olive was one year old, she began wellness Chiropractic care. Anna states, "I immediately began to see an improvement in her bowel regularity and sleep." Throughout the stages of development, Olive began developing some foot deviation as she walked. Through spinal and extremity adjustments, her feet have become more aligned and she was tripping less often. Olive loves being adjusted!

The Family: "My husband saw the added health benefits that Chiropractic care has on us girls and now he receives monthly wellness care, too. I love my healthier and happier family!"

Laura Stone, DC, MS
Family First Chiropractic Center
510 State Ave., Suite #3
Hampton, IL 61256
309-751-9790
Family1stchiropractic.com

Graham's Birth

Dr. Michael Southwick

Like most first-time moms to be, I was filled with a combination of excitement and anxiety. The downs of sickness and the ups of feeling the first flutter of movement; each day something new, and a day closer to meeting my miracle.

As the wife of a chiropractor, I wanted a natural birth, without interference. We discussed our wants and needs with our midwife, and created a beautiful birth plan.

I was due in January, so with the hustle and bustle of the holidays, my due date was fast approaching. On a beautiful Friday, late afternoon, I went into labor! It was perfect timing as my husband, Mike, had just finished with his last patient of the day.

Everything was progressing well; contractions were becoming stronger and more frequent. Soon it was time to push, and here is where the beautiful birth plan veered off course.

I dilated from three centimeters to ten centimeters in about ninety minutes, and I pushed for over three hours! The baby's heart rate began to fall. Our midwife told me I had ten minutes to deliver or they would have to use forceps. That was NOT what I wanted to hear! I prayed. I asked God to give me every ounce of strength I needed to deliver the baby. He answered my prayers. At 11:17 p.m. on January 14, Graham Larkin Southwick was born without forceps.

My birth plan was to have the baby immediately laid on my chest, but that didn't happen. Instead I saw Graham's head cradled in Mike's hands. I knew something was wrong when Mike was adjusting him IMMEDIATELY.

Graham's heart rate was falling because the cord was wrapped around his neck three times, and that is why pushing was so long. He was a yo-yo in the birth canal, and being strangled.

Everything in the delivery room was happening so fast—yet in slow motion. As Carol (our midwife) was removing the cord from around his neck, the delivery nurse was calling the NICU for a crash cart to intubate him—and my husband, my husband the chiropractor, let his innate take over. Mike felt and found the subluxation that was causing Graham to be grey and unresponsive. He adjusted him, and my baby screamed.

Graham cried, he began breathing, and turned from a dull grey to a lively pink. The nurse didn't even have a chance to complete her phone call.

The nurse hung up the phone and scooped up Graham and carried him across the room. She did a series of exams, checked his vitals, and gave him his Apgar score—a 10. He went from a 0 to a 10 in moments. Finally, I got to hold my son!

Our midwife and delivery nurse looked at Mike and said, "What did you do and how did you do it?" He answered by explaining Chiropractic to them!

I had always known the power of an adjustment, never doubted it. I can tell you, I have never been more thankful for that power and for my husband as I was in that moment. Graham is now a thriving sixteen-year-old—and still very well-adjusted!

Michael Southwick, DC and Amy Southwick
www.southwickchiropractic.com

Every Breath Matters

Dr. Nicole Lederman

I met Todd and his wife, Kristi, while working in Texas. Kristi was pregnant and I was given the honor of taking care of her throughout her pregnancy.

Kristi had a great pregnancy. She went along gracefully with a wonderful glow. Everyone expected the same for the delivery and the birth of their son. However, Jack was eager to meet his loving parents and decided he couldn't wait any longer. So, on February 20, Jack arrived six important weeks earlier than expected. (These final six weeks are huge to the development of an infant, especially for boys, whose lungs take a little longer to develop than girls'.)

Little Jack was an absolutely beautiful baby, with ten fingers and ten toes, cute ears, an adorable nose—he was ready to snuggle. There was just one problem: Jack was struggling to breathe.

His parents thought he just wasn't used to breathing yet. The doctors told them that his lungs were not done developing and every time he exhaled his lungs were collapsing.

Jack was rushed to another hospital equipped to deal with these serious problems and was placed on a respirator. He had a feeding tube, an IV, and a breathing tube. He was diagnosed with pulmonary hypertension, which is a big word that means "Your babe might not make it."

The doctors gave Jack surfactant and nitric oxide to help his lungs develop and get the much-needed oxygen to his body. Jack did beautifully for three days, when suddenly he stopped progressing and the doctors didn't have any answers for Jack's parents.

Todd and Kristi called me. I listened and gave some advice. I offered to come check Jack's spine and fragile nervous system, and adjust their son if I found cause to do so. They weren't sure; there was a lot of fear in the first couple of days. They talked about it, and then on a Saturday afternoon, I met Jack in the NICU. He was hooked up to many wires and wearing a "bili" mask under the lights.

The charts were graphing but this little boy was just lying there. I could only reach his neck, where I performed a focused exam of the upper-cervical spine and found his first neck bone to be subluxated to the left. I made a gentle contact and held it until it released. It was Jack's first adjustment. Five minutes later, Jack started kicking his legs like crazy; like he was waking up. You never know the power of the body! We were excited to see what would happen next.

The next day, the staff was amazed! Jack was doing better than expected, and his pulmonary hypertension resolved. They were calling him the miracle baby. Forty-eight hours later, the medical team removed all tubes and wires, and Jack was breathing on his own. He left the hospital within three weeks of birth—three weeks earlier than expected.

Jack is now a beautiful, healthy boy; living big and showing his brothers the way!

I am blessed to have played a part in Jack's story of health and recovery.

Dr. Nicole Lederman, a family chiropractor and certified acupuncturist, is in private practice at Awaken Chiropractic in Waterloo, Ontario, Canada. She specializes in preconception health, pre- and postnatal care, pediatrics, and women's health issues. Dr. Lederman has a passion for working with children and their families and for sharing her knowledge with her community and her fellow colleagues. She is an avid lecturer locally as well as internationally. Prior to sharing her passion in Waterloo, Dr. Nicole was an associate professor at Parker University where she taught Pediatrics, Chiropractic Technique, and Clinical Skills to the next generation of chiropractors. Contact Dr. Nicole via email or find her on Facebook.

Nicole Lederman, DC
Awaken Chiropractic
30 Dupont St. East, #105
Waterloo, ON N2J 2G9
awakenchiro.kw@gmail.com
www.awakenchirokw.com

Lessening Birth Trauma

Dr. Tana K. Frisina

Heather came to me when she was five months pregnant with Charlie. At that time, she looked like she was ready to give birth. Charlie was a large baby and Heather was just over five feet tall. Heather wanted to ensure she had as easy a delivery as possible; a friend recommended she seek Chiropractic care.

Heather did great under our care; yet, with only three weeks left before delivery, it was discovered that Charlie was in the breech position. I performed Webster's Technique on Heather and the next morning she had a sonogram that confirmed Charlie was head down and ready for delivery.

Unfortunately, even though he was in the correct position, Charlie had a huge head and Heather could not pass him through the birth canal. A C-Section was necessary for the safety of both child and mother. Heather remembers the doctor tugging on Charlie so hard the bed was moving.

Following his delivery, Charlie's sugar levels would not regulate, he would not breast feed, and he was jaundiced. Charlie spent nearly a week in Neonatal Intensive Care Unit (NICU) before finally being released.

After leaving the hospital, Heather came straight to my office, asking me to check little Charlie. He had several misalignments in his neck and the bones in his mouth were also out of alignment, most likely due to the birthing process. I gave Charlie his first Chiropractic adjustment and he went home.

The next day Heather called to say he was breast-feeding and had slept very well. She was so pleased that a Chiropractic treatment was able to help her experience the important bonding time associated with nursing her firstborn son.

Since his first adjustment, Charlie has been receiving Chiropractic care regularly for wellness and has been helped with sinus issues, earaches, hives, fevers, and all those bumps little boys have.

Heather has continued treatment and was able to have her second son, Lincoln, VBAC with no complications.

Lincoln had his first Chiropractic checkup two days after delivery and is a happy and healthy boy, just like his big brother.

Dr. Tana K. Frisina, is a Doctor of Chiropractic, who is Advanced Rated in Activator Methods, certified in the Webster Technique, as well as a certified whole food specialist. She has an extraordinary passion for helping families achieve a wellness lifestyle, whether through Chiropractic, therapies, nutrition and/or massage. Since opening in January 2013, The Frisina Family Wellness Center has offered more than 300 health and wellness seminars to assist the community in developing improved health.

Tana K. Frisina, DC
Frisina Family Wellness Center
1533 S. MacArthur Blvd.
Springfield, IL 62704
217-787-4345
www.frisinafamilychiropractic.com

A Happy Mother

Dr. Laura T. Brayton

Kristin was referred to my practice by her OB/
GYN after experiencing excruciating back pain that radiated
into her right leg. She had given birth via C-section eight
months prior due to the breech positioning of the baby and
was now having difficulty caring for her infant and herself due
to her back pain. Kristin's medical history indicated a spinal
surgery (a laminectomy) in her lower back, at the young age
of eighteen, following multiple sports injuries. The bottom two
vertebrae in her spine were also fused together during the surgery, therefore, creating altered biomechanics in her spine and
pelvis.

After a few Chiropractic sessions, her back pain lessened
tremendously and she decided to keep coming in for maintenance adjustments to keep feeling at her optimum. (I like
to call this mama self-care). Several months later, Kristin
announced she was pregnant with her second baby. We celebrated the news and she shared that she was hoping to have
as natural a childbirth experience as possible, considering that
she had a C-section the first time.

At times a VBAC (Vaginal Birth after Cesarean) is possible.
I saw Kristin once or twice per month until her third trimester,
at which time it was discovered that this baby was also in a
breech position. Our original excitement changed to disbelief
because it is rare for a woman to have two breech pregnancies.
I knew how badly Kristin wanted to experience a vaginal delivery, without medication or radical intervention; however, the
baby's position was definitely interfering with this plan.

The rest of the story is written in Kristin's own words:

"I would like to share my experience with my last pregnancy.

I went to Dr. Brayton for Webster Technique treatment at around thirty-two weeks, which is when I had just discovered the baby was still breech. I had hoped to avoid a repeat C-section (my first daughter was breech). After five weeks of regular treatments (three times per week), at thirty-eight weeks, my daughter finally turned. I was able to cancel my scheduled C-section and give birth to my second daughter vaginally and without the use of medication or other interventions. I arrived at the hospital 5 cm dilated at 1:45 p.m. and gave birth to Elisa at 3:19 p.m.! I owe my super-quick delivery to Dr. Brayton's regular adjustments.

"I highly recommend this treatment, especially if you are hoping for a natural, vaginal delivery."

What a thrill it was for me to be involved in supporting Kristin and her new child through this process. Avoiding a C-section was not only great for Kristin, but also exceptional for the newborn baby who entered the world the way we were meant to enter.

Laura T. Brayton, DC, CACCP
Hoboken Chiropractic + Wellness, Inc.
50 Harrison St., Suite 316
Hoboken, NJ 07030
201-792-3544
www.HobokenChiro.com

Birth Trauma

Dr. Peter Amlinger

I first met Michael when he was just over two months old. A patient who attended the orientation class I hold in my office for new clients shared what he had learned with Michael's father. He told him that Michael's ability to heal was far greater than he had been led to believe and that all children should be checked for subluxations as soon after birth as possible. It was only because this information was shared that Michael found himself in a Chiropractic office.

Michael had a difficult start to life. At eight and a half pounds, he was a big baby. While coming down the birth canal, his shoulder got stuck. To overcome the shoulder dystocia, the attending doctor used vacuum extraction. He had to apply it twice because it slipped off the first time. When Michael arrived, he was blue and his breathing rate was very rapid. His initial Apgar score was 4. Mom doesn't know what the five-minute Apgar was because he had been whisked away to neonatal intensive care.

It was determined that due to the forces used in his birth process, the phrenic nerve (nerve controlling the diaphragm for breathing) had been completely avulsed. It had been torn from its origin. The result was that the right side of Michael's diaphragm was completely paralyzed, making it impossible to oxygenate his blood. To assist, he was fitted for a neonatal CPAP (Continuous Positive Airway Pressure) unit to drive oxygen into his blood.

The diaphragm also acts as a valve, especially in newborns, to keep food in the stomach. Due to the paralysis, this functional valve was nonexistent and Michael could not keep food down; he was diagnosed with gastroesophageal reflux disease

(GERD). He would belch, wretch, and vomit. Therefore, he was put on omeprazole and domperidone, two potent drugs (not tested for safety in newborns) in an attempt to control the reflux symptoms. His feeding difficulties negatively impacted his growth, so a nasogastric feeding tube was installed soon after birth. It was still in place when I first met him. Even with the feeding tube, Michael could only be given small amounts of food at a time and he regurgitated most of it.

Michael had spent the first six weeks of his life at Toronto's Sick Children's Hospital. The attending physicians told his parents that the diaphragm would always be paralyzed and that the pull from the normal muscular action on his left side would create a large distortion in his posture. The nerve supply to his right arm was also compromised.

They said there was little or no hope for improvement. They suggested placating his diaphragm, which would have meant pinning it down into the position it should have been in. Because it was paralyzed, it was stuck motionless way up in his chest cavity. The physicians were not sure what doing this procedure would do for him. Mom and Dad chose to refuse this intervention.

Michael was sent home, underweight, with a very rapid heart rate, feeding tube installed with little food going in, and reflux disease.

It was then when my patient, who worked with Michael's father, told him about Chiropractic:

> "My chiropractor taught me that your son's capacity to heal is far greater than you have been led to believe. Many children suffer from this thing called a subluxation, and my chiropractor sees a ton of children. Maybe you should take your son to see him."

Michael's parents were anxious to try anything to help their son; so they scheduled a Chiropractic assessment for him. I met Michael on Friday, November 11, 2011. In my thirty years of Chiropractic practice and teaching Chiropractic around the world, I have never examined anyone with a more severe atlas subluxation. The top vertebra in Michael's tiny neck was subluxated to the right.

We explained to Mom and Dad that Chiropractic does not treat or cure anything; it doesn't focus on what's wrong with a person, but rather works to release what is perfect within all of us, our inborn capacity to heal. Our focus, if they chose to accept care, would be to check Michael's nervous system for subluxation-induced nerve interference and then to remove it with a specific Chiropractic adjustment. Mom was eager to start care on the first visit, so we did.

On Monday of the following week, Michael came in for his second visit. Mom was ecstatic. After only one Chiropractic adjustment, the retching and reflux stopped, and Mom chose to discontinue the drugs for reflux. We continued to check Michael three times per week.

After two weeks of care, the feeding tube was no longer necessary and was removed. Michael was eating normal amounts of formula and keeping it all down. He was also starting to grow!

After one month of adjustments, a follow-up ultrasound revealed that the right-sided diaphragmatic paralysis was completely resolved, and the left and right sides of the diaphragm were working perfectly together.

Within three months of starting care, Michael's arm movement normalized and he caught up on all his developmental milestones! We continued to check him and he walked on time. Today, he is a perfectly normal, four-year-old boy who is learning how to play hockey.

This wonderful example of our innate ability to heal and the power of Chiropractic with respect to releasing that healing power has left me with two questions that drive my passion to educate as many people as I can about the premise that Chiropractic is based on. Life flows over the nervous system and it, and only it, heals as long as there is no interference. Chiropractic detects and removes interference with the adjustment. The questions are:

1. *Why did the physicians at Sick Children's Hospital not detect Michael's subluxation?*

   The answer is simple: they have no training to do so. Only chiropractors are trained to detect and correct subluxations.

2. *How many children are lying in hospital beds or living compromised lives because no one ever told their parents about the wonders of Chiropractic?*

I am thankful that I was blessed to be Michael's chiropractor. I am also thankful that my patient had the knowledge and cared enough about others to share what he knew about Chiropractic.

Peter Amlinger, DC
210-3476 Glen Erin Drive
Mississauga, Ontario Canada L5l 3R4
905-569-7080
dr.peteramlinger@me.com

Answering the Call

Dr. Paul Blumsack

The ringing of our home phone awakened me. Glassy-eyed, I looked at the clock and wondered who on earth would be calling me at four thirty in the morning. For a moment, I thought of ignoring it, but something in my spirit told me to answer the call. "Good morning, this is Paul."

"Hi, Paul. This is John. Our son was just born a few minutes ago and you were right about the doctor's pulling, tugging, and twisting on our son's neck during the delivery. We want to see when you can come and check him."

"Congratulations, John. How is your son doing?"

"He seems to be fine, from what I can tell."

"Tell you what, I have office hours this morning, starting at eight thirty, and I break for lunch at twelve thirty. I will come and check him during my break. Okay?"

"Sounds good to me. I'll see you then."

I hung up the phone and was going to return to bed for another hour when I felt the spirit once again prompt me, this time to check this little boy now. I called the hospital and asked the front desk to call down to their room. John answered the phone. "Hey John, this is Paul. I'm on my way now to check your son. I will be there in about thirty minutes."

"Thanks, Paul. I'll see you then."

I drove to the hospital. When I walked into the room, I was introduced to this precious newborn. I asked permission from his mother to check him and she said yes.

On observation, I noticed his head was turned to one side. In checking his range of motion, I noticed that whenever I tried to move his head to the center or to the opposite side, his head would turn back to the favored side. I did this several times to confirm my findings. Both Mom and Dad could see this as well. I then checked the first vertebra in his neck to see if it was subluxated (misaligned), and it was. This typically puts pressure on the brainstem, which affects the body's ability to function and heal properly.

Subluxations, or misalignments, present at the first vertebra in the neck are common in most newborns as the current "modern birth procedures" create stress on the baby's head, neck, and shoulders.

Using the tip of my pinky, I gently applied some light pressure on his subluxated first vertebra and gave him his first adjustment. It glided smoothly back into place. I then rechecked him and he no longer favored that one side. His head was moving easily. I told Mom and Dad that he would be fine and that I would recheck him later that night. I left and headed to my practice.

I called John at lunchtime to see how everyone was doing and I was told their son had been placed in the Neonatal Intensive Care Unit for having a hole in his lung. Apparently the doctor at the time of delivery noticed something out of the ordinary and immediately ordered tests. The results came back mid-morning. I asked John what the doctors were planning on doing. He said, "Nothing. The doctors told us that all we can do is wait and see if the body will heal itself."

This statement floored me because this is what we teach our patients every day in our practice. The body has the ability to heal itself as long as there is no interference. Several days later, this is exactly what happened. Having been cleared of the interference at his brainstem, his little body healed itself and he was released from the hospital. Twenty years later, he is still under my Chiropractic care and living a healthy and vibrant life.

I am so glad I answered the call!

Paul Blumsack, DC
Blumsack Family Chiropractic
3770 Due West Rd., Suite 200
Marietta, GA 30064
770-362-6430
www.blumsackfamilychiropractic.com
Live Better ... Live Longer

Happy Birthday

Dr. Tim Young

It was a Tuesday afternoon when my assistant, Kresha, handed me a phone message from one of my patients. Mark and his wife, Christy, had recently become patients in our office and were excited about the expected birth of their first child. I adjusted Christy for the usual hip misalignments and neck issues that often come along with pregnancy. Mark was a former professional wrestler, now pastor, who "Needed to be adjusted from head to toe."

The message asked me to call Mark as soon as possible. There had been complications with the delivery and he wanted to ask me some questions. During a break, I called Mark on his cell phone. When he answered, it was very obvious he was extremely upset and stressed. Mark explained that he and Christy had decided to have a home birth. During the delivery, their son, Coleman, became "stuck" in the birth canal. They later found out that Coleman was a ten-pound baby and Christy was not physically made for such an undertaking. They immediately rushed to the hospital where medical intervention quickly began.

Mark's voice began to shake as he explained that Coleman was in ICU and not doing well. His heart rate was extremely elevated and his respiration rate was so low it seemed like he was barely breathing. Mark then explained that the doctors were unsure of the cause of his altered vitals. Even worse, they didn't know what to do to help him. Mark asked me if there was anything I could do.

My first thought was to tell him I was on my way, but the fact that Coleman was in a hospital posed a real problem. I told Mark that the only way I could possibly see Coleman is if the pediatrician on call approved it. We both knew the odds of that were slim to none. At this point in my life, I was forty-two years old and had been in practice for about fifteen years. I had experienced enough personal situations to know that the hand of God is in all things, but what happened next, in my mind, was a great example of what is possible.

I have patients from all professions and walks of life. They drive from across town, across the street, or from three hours away. I have thousands of patients on file, but only one patient is a pediatrician. In all the hospitals in Oklahoma City, on all the floors, in all the rooms, and all the babies being born, guess who was on the floor at the time Mark called to see if he could get me cleared to see Coleman? You guessed it, my patient. The odds were staggering.

When Mark explained to the pediatrician that he and his wife would like for me to come to the hospital and see if I could help in any way, the doctor said that he would make sure I got in. The doctor explained that at this point anything Dr. Young could do would be greatly welcomed.

I left my office that Tuesday just after 6:00 p.m. and headed to the hospital. When I arrived at the ICU front desk, there were three nurses waiting on me. I didn't even get my name out when one of the nurses said, "You must be Uncle Tim. We have been waiting on you."

Within minutes, I had blue scrubs on, booties on my feet, and a silly little cloth hat on my head. I then rushed into one of the most sterile and cold environments I have ever seen. As I looked around the room, I immediately noticed Mark and Christy standing, looking over at a plastic bed containing their little angel; tubes, wires, and monitors hooked up to him. It was a scene right out of a bad science-fiction movie.

I walked over to the new parents to get more information, and I was immediately struck by what I saw. When I looked into Christy's eyes, the white was gone, only blood red. This poor girl looked like she had been hit by a train and was exhausted.

I turned to Mark and asked what had happened. Mark said that when they arrived at the hospital, Coleman was stuck in the birth canal. "They pushed him back in, turned his head, and ripped him out." The level of pressure on Christy was so great that it burst every blood vessel in her eyes.

I remember taking a deep breath and calming myself before looking at Coleman. The image of what Mark had just told me was more than I was used to and to see that much pain in someone's eyes was unsettling. Knowing Christy as well as I do, I believe the pain I was seeing wasn't as much from the physical trauma as it was from the fact that her baby boy was lying in a bundle of wires and she couldn't hold him.

As I walked to the incubator, I looked up and noticed wires leading to a monitor. There were several different numbers, words, and beeps coming from the monitor that I didn't really pay attention to or would I have known what they meant. But, there were two numbers in particular that I did understand and knew very well that they were not appropriate for a newborn.

At the time, I didn't fully recognize the significance of what was happening. If I had, I would have taken notes and documented everything in better detail, but I was not there to document. I do not remember the exact numbers, but I can say that Coleman's heart rate was going crazy and his respiration rate was so low you could barely see his chest move.

When I looked down at Coleman for the first time, I had to stop and take another deep breath. Coleman's little eyes were as blood-red as his mother's. The amount of force this little man had been under was hard for me to wrap my mind around. Without hesitation, I reached through the wires and gently moved Coleman to a seated position facing away from me. With my thumbs I began to palpate his tiny spine until I reached the seventh thoracic rib head on the right, which was protruding out so far you could physically see it. I took my right thumb and precisely set the rib back to its normal position.

After I finished palpating the rest of his spine, I laid Coleman on his back, head toward me, and began to palpate his neck. I found his atlas to be rotated very far to the right. Very gently, but with great intent, I adjusted his atlas, returning it to its intended position. I then returned Coleman back to his original lying position and removed my hands. I stood quietly and waited for any immediate response. I did not expect what happened next.

Coleman took a deep breath and seemed to immediately relax. The monitor that Coleman was hooked up to started to change. Me, four nurses, and Coleman's parents watched as his heart rate came down and his respiration slowly returned to normal. We all stood in silence, in awe of what was happening.

The silence was suddenly broken by one of the nurses, who was very upset I was there. Standing in the back of the room with her arms crossed, she said, "Those machines are not that reliable."

No one even responded. I wanted to ask her why, if the machine was so unreliable, do you stand around and worship it? I decided that it wasn't worth the argument. I gave Mark and Christy a hug and told them that Coleman would be fine; then I left the hospital and went home.

The next day, the pediatrician who made it possible for me to see Coleman, came to my office to get adjusted. He said, "I don't know what you did, but Coleman is going home today."

I get asked by patients to attend many birthday parties, graduations, and weddings. I usually decline due to the fact if I started going to them I would be at some event every day. However, when I was invited to attend Coleman's first birthday party, I felt it was important that I go.

When my wife and I showed up at the church where the party was being held, we couldn't believe how many people were there. We had never seen that many people show up for a child's birthday party. Like us, they must have felt that this party was special. I was also amazed by how many patients of mine were there. Then, it occurred to me, that they were all referred, directly or indirectly, by Mark and Christy.

As the party moved on, my wife and I enjoyed talking with everyone and hearing their stories about how much Chiropractic had helped them and their kids. Mark then took a microphone and asked if he could have everyone's attention. He thanked everyone for coming, then he said, "Before we have some cake, I would like to say the blessing, but before I do, I would like to say, God bless Dr. Young for saving our Coleman and God bless Chiropractic."

As I sit here and write this story, my eyes tear up and I feel the emotion I felt that day. There wasn't a dry eye at the party, and the celebration of a little boy's first birthday took on a whole new meaning.

Mark and Christy now have three boys, and they all come in for their adjustments on a regular basis. All three are well adjusted, unvaccinated, and extremely healthy. I love this family dearly and I tell this story often.

I have been told that this story is nothing more than an anecdote and it has no validity because there is no evidence to prove what happened. My response is always the same: It's not anecdotal to Coleman or his parents, and they are the only ones who matter.

As the developer of chiropractic, Dr. B. J. Palmer once said:

"We never know how far-reaching something we may say, think, or do today will affect the lives of millions tomorrow."

Tim Young, DC
www.youngchiropracticokc.com

Cooper's Story

Dr. Wanda Lee MacPhee
Dr. Andrew Kleinknecht

There are few things more stressful for parents than having a baby with health challenges. Mylene enjoyed a healthy pregnancy. With Chiropractic care during those nine months, the new mom-to-be was in wonderful condition for the birth of her first child.

Things, however, did not go as easily in the delivery room. Cooper experienced a number of challenges at birth resulting from a rare and undetected congenital deficiency. Considering the trauma and difficulties that his little body experienced, it was a miracle he survived. Clearly Cooper was determined to be here, and he was fortunate to have the emergency care that allowed him to live through his first hours and days on earth.

After he was stabilized, his parents were given the green light to take their baby home. Shortly thereafter, Cooper was in our office for his first Chiropractic checkup. He was already two months old.

Upon examination, it was clear there were significant subluxations (spinal displacements affecting normal function) that were preventing him from being fully healthy. Chiropractic care would certainly be beneficial for this infant.

Unfortunately, other health care providers on Cooper's team did not support Chiropractic, leaving Mylene and her husband, Bernie, to choose between great medical care and their desire to give Cooper every possible helping hand. These new parents were put in the unfortunate position to forfeit Chiropractic care in order to work with the hospital program that was also essential for his well-being.

Fast forward two years and the completion of the hospital program, at last! This young family was now free to return to Chiropractic for help. Despite the specialized hospital program, Mylene and Bernie had lingering concerns about Cooper's health. He was not walking and unable to sit upright. Cooper was underweight and reaching developmental milestones more appropriate for a ten- or eleven-month-old than a toddler. Despite his medical care, it was clear to all of us that Cooper was not functioning at his full potential.

Scans, examinations, and a review of Cooper's medical files showed us a number of subluxation patterns that were likely contributing to Cooper's lack of progress in sitting, walking, and ability to thrive. He may not have been able to speak for himself, but he had no trouble communicating where things felt good and where things felt bad! Cooper immediately loved his adjustments and would happily sit on my lap and lean into the areas that he wanted me to check out!

After only three weeks of Chiropractic care, Cooper was able to hold his head up and sit straighter.

In a few more weeks, he was starting to move and scoot around the floor. Over the next few months, we added craniosacral therapy and then a pediatric physiotherapist to Cooper's team. The progress of his structure and nerve system function continued.

It was so exciting to see him progress and begin to thrive—putting on weight, sleeping a bit better, and beginning to verbalize!

A few short months later, Cooper is on the move, scooting and crawling around the floor.

A year later, Cooper is able to walk unassisted.

Fast forward two years, and he is starting school, playing on the playground, and climbing up on the table for his adjustments. Cooper sets a great example of enjoying the experience and getting the most benefit from his Chiropractic care!

There is no greater compliment than having parents trust you with their baby.

This is even truer for those children with special needs. We know this is the ultimate in confidence, and we relish the opportunity to assist the next generation to be even healthier.

Chiropractic care offers the opportunity to positively

impact children as their bodies and nerve patterns develop, and movement habits and postures are being formed. This is the time when correction is both simplest and most revealing on a lifetime of health and well-being.

Wanda Lee MacPhee BSc, DC
Andrew Kleinknecht BSc, DC
St Margaret's Bay Chiropractic Centre
5715 St Margaret's Bay Road
Nova Scotia, Canada B3Z 2E3
902-826-1088
info@stmargaretsbaychiro.com
www.stmargaretsbaychiro.com

Delivery of Jamie

Dr. Wendy Coburn

I have so many amazing patient birth stories I could share, but I am actually going to share my own. Jamie is our third child. When it came time for him to come into the world, we were so excited.

Our first child was born two weeks early; our second two weeks late; and Jamie, we figured, would be right on time. (Just so you know, they all came exactly at the time they were supposed to.) As a chiropractor and Chiropractic patient, I receive wellness care: weekly Chiropractic care to ensure my nervous system is optimally functioning at all times. This was the case during my pregnancy, to help this precious baby grow strong and free of subluxations and stress.

I had finished my last shift. As I played with our twenty-three-month-old and thirteen-month-old, I excitedly awaited Jamie's arrival. Like with our two other children, my labor started when I was asleep. From ten p.m. or so, I quietly labored through the night, knowing not to disturb anyone, recognizing that labor is a journey and we had some time. So, I had a good sleep.

When eight a.m. rolled around, my two children jumped into our bed and immediately my labor stopped. I went the entire day with nothing more happening. As a chiropractor, who fully understands the human body, and having had two other children, I knew not to worry. Nevertheless, I was anxious and excited, and wondered when labor would begin again.

By noon, I called a colleague and asked if she would come over and check me. She adjusted my sacrum and upper-cervical spine with an activator, a very light method of adjusting. It was like a light switch was turned on because within twenty minutes, my labor started again. I was readjusted and within another twenty minutes I was in active labor.

The time span from my first adjustment to the birth of our wonderful son, was a short two hours. Jamie was born under-water—a stress-free birth. Given the right environment, with removal of any interferences, this wonderful machine we call the human body can adapt and adjust quickly given the right messages.

> Chiropractic is essential for pregnancy and delivery; not to mention postnatal for mom and baby.

After having firsthand experience on the value of regular Chiropractic care during pregnancy, I feel completely compe-tent and informed to suggest Chiropractic for every pregnant woman.

Wendy Coburn, DC
West Edmonton Family Chiropractic Studio
780-484-2272
www.chiropracticbalance.com

From C-Section to Healthy Delivery

Dr. Denise Scott

Many women daydream and plan the story of their life from a young age, and many of those dreams include starting a family. As a child, you see life through rose-colored glasses; everything thing is perfect like in the movies—then reality hits! This is what happened to Naomi when she found out she was pregnant. She was excited to learn she was expecting her first child and began thinking of baby names and nursery themes. Everything was as peachy as she had hoped—until delivery time.

She was admitted into the hospital and then the terror began. She was induced and the medical model thwarted her plans of having a natural home birth. When it was all said and done, she had a traumatic Caesarian birth, leaving her with feelings of regret and remorse. Thankfully, with time, wounds are healed.

I met Naomi when she was pregnant with her second child. Her baby, Sarah, was in a breech position and due in two weeks. Her options were a C-section or an external cephalic version per her birth provider. When Naomi asked about Chiropractic, her birth provider told her that at thirty-eight weeks Chiropractic was not effective. Naomi refused to have the same experience she had with her first delivery; so out of desperation, she did some research. She found that Chiropractic can help, especially the Webster Technique.

I am a certified Webster provider and I was the closest provider to Naomi; so she came to me for help.

When Naomi came into the office for her first visit, she was full of questions and very nervous. I patiently answered all concerns and eased her fears. She decided to give Chiropractic a try. I began adjusting Naomi with the Webster Technique every day until her next appointment with her midwife on Thursday. I told Naomi to give me a call after her appointment, with the results of the baby's position. I did not receive a call Thursday; so out of concern, I sent a text to ask what the verdict was. Naomi had delivered baby Sarah naturally Thursday evening and was already back in the comfort of her home, enjoying her new baby!!!

I was excited and shocked at the same time. We chatted for a while and she told me her husband wanted to come in because he hurt himself during delivery. She did all the work and he needed the adjustment!

I cannot take credit for making her baby move into the proper position, the wisdom of her body allowed the shift to occur. I can only be grateful for the opportunity to serve with the skill and knowledge I obtained in school. I now have some work to do to share how Chiropractic can help optimize the space in the pregnant pelvis and increase the chances for the proper birth position to birth providers in my community.

Every woman deserves the right to experience the birth she desires and Chiropractic care during pregnancy definitely increases the chances.

Denise Scott, DC
Circle of Healing Chiropractic
215 Dalton Drive, Suite C
Desoto, Texas 75115
214-628-1952
www.circleofhealingchiro.com

Failed IVF to Baby!

Dr. Brenda Fairchild

Lisa came into my office somewhat reluctantly; a little unsure; and in a sad, vulnerable state. She had been trying for over three years to have a baby, to no avail. She had suffered multiple miscarriages.

She heard through the grapevine that I had helped many women have a baby. She was nervous about Chiropractic care and what she had seen on TV—but she was desperate and willing to try anything.

During one entire year, she attempted to get pregnant naturally and had one miscarriage.

Over the next two years, they did three rounds of IUI (Intrauterine insemination); not one pregnancy resulted. She then had two rounds of IVF (in vitro fertilization). Each IVF cycle produced a pregnancy, but both ended in heartbreaking miscarriages.

The fertility clinic wanted to set her up for a third round but she decided to take a break. This long, arduous, unsuccessful process led Lisa to my office.

> She could get pregnant, but could not sustain a pregnancy. She was frustrated and looking for answers.

On her exam, a few things were noted. She had extremely poor posture from a desk job she had worked at for years. Her shoulders were rolled forward, the right shoulder was higher than the left; her right hip was rolled forward, mimicking a scoliosis, even though she did not have a history of scoliosis. Her muscles were very tight and dehydrated.

Lisa also had misalignments of her sacrum, her lumbar

spine (especially L3 and 4), along with misalignments in her upper-cervical neck area.

She was experiencing headaches three to four times a week, and irregular bowel function. It was not uncommon for her to evacuate only once or twice a week.

She mentioned being involved in several minor car accidents, but had never gone to the hospital or doctor following these mishaps.

Her menstrual periods were sporadic, brown to black in color, accompanied by lots of clots and painful cramping. One of the doctors told her she had polycystic ovary syndrome (PCOS), but she wasn't convinced.

She also said that her sleep patterns were horrible. Most days, she would awaken around 3:00 a.m. and be unable to get back to sleep. She thought it had to do with the medication and hormones she had been on. She also admitted her diet wasn't the best, but was trying to be proactive in changing her intake.

Over the next few months, we worked on improving her posture with the Chiropractic adjustments and I also incorporated using The Webster Technique. This specific adjustment focuses on the lumbar spine and pelvic bones, as well as the muscles and ligaments in those areas.

The goal is to balance and maintain the maternal pelvis.

On several occasions, I also checked her entire spine and performed adjustments as indicated on examination. We did make a few changes in her diet, and I suggested some vitamins and minerals as well.

Within the first month of Chiropractic care, her headaches were no longer a part of her life. She was sleeping through the night and her period was red with minimal clots and cramping. She was moving her bowels on a regular basis. She was one incredibly happy woman.

I continued to work with Lisa over the next few months, until one day she came in and said she was six weeks pregnant—no IUI or IVF.

This pregnancy occurred naturally. She was still a little nervous because she had not carried a baby past twelve weeks.

Well ... I am happy to report that Lisa and her husband welcomed a beautiful, healthy baby girl, Chloe, into their lives, making their family whole!

She did it!! Today, Lisa is pregnant with her second baby, who was also conceived naturally.

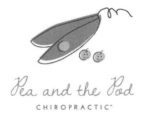

Pea and the Pod
CHIROPRACTIC

Brenda Fairchild, DC, CACCP
Pea and the Pod Chiropractic
One Centurian Dr., Suite 104
Newark, DE 19713
302-455-PEAS (7327)
www.peapodchiro.com
Specialized in Fertility, Women's Health, Pregnancy, and Pediatrics

Painful Pregnancy

Dr. Dina Sgambati

In June 2014, a patient presented for Chiropractic care in her thirty-second week of pregnancy. Not only was her baby breech, but she was also suffering from strong, stabbing back pain as well. It had become impossible for her to bend over or even stand up from a chair without wincing from the pain. Her daily walks around the pier had been reduced to hobbling a fraction of the distance. Each step felt more like a limp as she attempted to get where she needed to go.

She felt discouraged and frustrated trying to exercise in an effort to keep her weight in check and safeguard her health after being given a diagnosis of gestational diabetes. Sometimes anxiety would set in because she didn't know exactly what was wrong or how to fix it.

> Oftentimes she would give up, resign herself to her limitations, and think, "I guess it's normal to have pain during pregnancy. People told me my back would hurt."

As she began to seek out solutions, work colleagues and a local lactation consultant recommended physical therapy and/or Chiropractic. Ultimately, she took the advice of her sister, who wholeheartedly endorsed Chiropractic care.

An Internet search led her to our office. She was so excited to find a chiropractor who specialized in caring for maternity patients. She was filled with hope and a knowingness that "this was meant to be."

During her initial examination, I performed an analysis of her pelvis utilizing the Webster Technique. Subluxation of the right sacro-iliac (SI) joint coupled with a left tilt of sacral apex had caused instability of the pelvis. Compensatory changes resulted in an imbalance of the muscles and ligaments of the pelvis, as well as subluxations in other regions of the spine.

I performed several gentle adjustments, prescribed a stabilization belt, and applied ice on the inflamed SI joint. The patient noticed a significant improvement the very first night.

I applied the necessary adjustments two more times that week in order to restore pelvic alignment and reduce intrauterine constraint. At the end of her first week of Chiropractic care, an ultrasound revealed that the baby had flipped into a normal head-down position. We were all so excited to hear the news!

Subsequent checkups with her OB/GYN confirmed the baby's head-down position right up until the day of delivery.

The patient continued to receive Chiropractic care each week for the remainder of her pregnancy. She reported that she was walking four times around the pier each day, maintaining her weight, and enjoying the last few weeks of bonding time with her young daughter.

Within hours after the birth of her son, the patient was walking around with ease. Her husband marveled as she easily bent down to get something from her bag and said, "Wow! You weren't able to do that after the birth of our daughter."

She experienced firsthand that feeling good during pregnancy is not only normal, but attainable through Chiropractic care.

Dr. Sgambati, a prenatal chiropractor and mother of two, has pursued advanced training to establish a maternity specialty. She is an active member of the American Pregnancy Association, International Chiropractic Pediatric Association, and Webster Technique certified. A contributing writer for many publications, including the *North Jersey Expectant Mother's Guide*, *Hoboken Digest*, and *Hoboken Family Alliance Newsletter*; Dr. Sgambati was also honored to participate in the award-winning documentary Orgasmic Birth alongside many world-renowned birth experts.

Dina Sgambati, DC
Priority Chiropractic
Hoboken, NJ
www.prioritychironj.com

The Value of Prenatal Care

Dr. DoniBeth Davis

I began seeing a twenty-seven-year-old woman for neck pain and numbness in her hands, bilaterally. About six months after starting Chiropractic care, she became pregnant. At that time, she had experienced significant relief of her initial complaints and was being seen on a maintenance frequency.

She continued with Chiropractic care throughout her pregnancy. She was able to stay relatively comfortable, with minimal to no back pain; although the symptoms in her hands returned during pregnancy.

It was determined by her birth provider that the baby needed to be delivered via Cesarean section. She had a scheduled date for delivery and asked if I would come to the hospital to check her daughter right away after delivery. The surgery went as scheduled, although the doctor had to use a vacuum to extract her from the uterus, which added significant increased pressure on the baby's spine.

I was able to get to the hospital within five hours of delivery and examine the baby. At that time, she had not had a bowel movement. I found restriction in the top and bottom of her spine (C1 and sacrum) and provided an appropriate adjustment to the joints right there in the hospital.

Within the next twenty-four hours, she began having bowel movements regularly. This was a second child and her mother was not able to successfully breast feed her first child. Now, she was able to breast feed without any issues for either herself or the baby.

Prior to giving birth, the mother had said this would be her last pregnancy. However, within a few short weeks of caring for her easygoing newborn, she said she was reconsidering her decision because it had been such an easy transition with the new baby. The baby had a very happy temperament.

> I have consistently seen that mothers who have Chiropractic care during pregnancy also have babies that are easier to care for and have a smooth transition into life outside of the womb.

It is a great example of a how the baby is positively affected from the mother having less stress on her nervous system and full expression of life. In this scenario, despite having an unnatural delivery, care during pregnancy and immediately following delivery allowed for the newborn to adapt quickly and easily.

DoniBeth Davis, DC
Sozo Chiropractic
3720 72nd Avenue
Kenosha, WI 53144
262-764-9301

How Past Injuries Affect Your Life

Dr. Kareen Oosterhart

Growing up, I had my fair share of injuries. As a child, I had a riding lawn mower tip over on top of me when I was sitting on it, twice. Each time, I was fortunate enough to not break any bones.

As a teenager I worked at a local pizza shop. I did everything from making pizzas to delivering them. One winter evening, I borrowed my mom's SUV to make deliveries. Unfortunately, it was no match against the slick roads, and I slid her SUV down a nine-foot ditch, up the embankment, and into a tree. I was slammed into the middle console, with my seat belt on, and back into the driver's seat as the SUV landed in the ditch. Although I sustained no broken bones, I believe the problems I faced later originated from this accident.

The occasional migraines I had been having, became more frequent and intense around that time. I almost did not graduate high school due to so many missed days caused by migraines. Thankfully, I had some amazing people on my side who witnessed firsthand my struggles with migraines. They fought for me to walk that stage with my classmates.

The worst outcome of my accidents, though, came after high school, when I met and later married my husband.

We had been married for a couple years and decided to start a family. My husband and I tried for over a year and a half to become pregnant, and were unsuccessful. When I interviewed with a chiropractor for a massage therapist position, we decided to wait a while before trying to get pregnant again.

Soon after the job interview, I began Chiropractic care with Doctor Kareen Oosterhart. Two weeks after my first adjustment, my husband and I were blessed with the most amazing news: not only did I receive the position, I was also pregnant!

> I believe the adjustments corrected my pelvis and the subluxations in my spine, allowing my body to carry a healthy, beautiful baby boy.

Chiropractic care has also given that beautiful baby boy a better chance at survival, with a thriving immune system after being one month premature.

He is now four years old, healthy, and regularly adjusted! And we have also just welcomed a second miracle baby boy!

Along with the miracles of my two boys, I can thankfully say that my migraines have also greatly diminished and are significantly less intense as they once were.

My family and I owe so much to Chiropractic care! Without it, I do not believe I would have the pleasure and blessings of being a mommy!

Kareen Oosterhart, DC
Village Chiropractic Wellness Center, P.L.C.
798 W. Mile Rd.
Kalkaska, MI 49646
231-258-4023
www.village-chiropractic.com

In Dire Need at Thirty-Six Weeks

Dr. Maggie Hunsicker

I am no stranger to Chiropractic care. I had been seeing a chiropractor semi-regularly over the last ten years. Pregnancy brain does strange things though, and I did not find Dr. Maggie until I needed her when I was thirty-six weeks pregnant with baby number four.

Linden's pregnancy was my fourth in eight years and my body needed help getting Linden into an optimal position. She had been flipping back and forth to a breech position for weeks. I contacted Dr. Maggie in desperation, as I had tried many other ways to get Linden into a head-down position so that I could achieve a natural, vaginal birth.

When I meet Dr. Maggie for the first time, it was instant love. She made me feel safe and supported, listened to my history, and asked more than the generic questions a first-time visit typically brings. We chatted for over an hour and I instantly felt safe in Dr. Maggie's care.

Dr. Maggie was able to identify what was going on within my body that was causing my baby to prefer a breech position. Since Linden was breech at thirty-six weeks and my body had been growing her in a not so optimal alignment for the first eight months, I started seeing Dr. Maggie on a continual basis. Mondays, Wednesdays, and Fridays were my Dr. Maggie trips.

The right side of my torso was so tight it was causing my belly to grow lopsided. I could tell that Linden preferred the left side of my uterus versus the right. After a few adjustments with Dr. Maggie, my body was starting to even out and my right side was not so tight. By the middle of my thirty-eighth week, Linden had positioned herself head down!

Dr. Maggie had worked on getting my pelvis to open up and

my muscles and ligaments to release enough for Linden to do so comfortably. I believe this is why Linden was able to move down and get comfortable in a head-down position.

When I went into labor Linden, I was worried about Linden getting in a posterior position. Dr. Maggie came over to my house, gave me an adjustment, and stayed for a few hours to make sure Linden stayed in a good position. I felt so taken care of and loved!

After having Linden, Dr. Maggie came over to our home for Linden's first adjustment. I will never forget that sweet, special time. From being breech for so long inside of me, Linden had some compression issues from the pressure that the breech position put on her little head and neck.

Over the next six months, Dr. Maggie helped work that out on Linden and also helped me get back into optimal health, with plenty of postpartum adjustments and constant encouragement to be healthy.

I cannot imagine what the end of my last pregnancy, labor, and postpartum period would have looked like without Dr. Maggie's Chiropractic care!

Dr. Maggie received her certification in Chiropractic Pediatrics with the International Chiropractic Pediatric Association and is also Webster Technique Certified. She has a strong affection for pregnancy and pediatric patients but believes that Chiropractic care is essential for all ages. As a fourth-generation graduate from Palmer College of Chiropractic, Dr. Maggie is dedicated to encourage, educate, and inspire individuals to incorporate Chiropractic care into their lifestyle.

Maggie Hunsicker, DC
www.drmaggieh.com

Premature Labor

Dr. Paul Blumsack

I was in my first year of Chiropractic school when my wife, Paula, announced that she was pregnant with our second child. We hoped this pregnancy would be easier than her first, when she developed toxemia. She had to have an induced labor and was not able to hold the baby until her blood pressure lowered to a safe level; this took three days—probably the longest three days of her life.

Paula's pregnancy progressed well until the twenty-seventh week, when she started having severe contractions. We called the OB/GYN's office and Paula was immediately scheduled for an office visit. Upon examination, Paula was told that she was in premature labor. Her cervix had started to dilate and her only option was medication and bed rest for the remainder of the pregnancy; otherwise there was a high risk of losing the baby.

Reluctantly we chose to have Paula start taking the medication. The contractions stopped temporarily but the side effects made Paula feel tired all the time. In addition, her heart kept fluttering.

In reading the pamphlet provided with the medication, the side effects she was experiencing were definitely from the medication. And we also read that what she was taking was as an asthma medication—and actually contraindicated for pregnant women. Scared of what we read, Paula stopped taking the medication to avoid any risk to her and to our unborn son.

Her contractions returned; so we were in a race against time to find a safer, natural option. I decided to call my chiropractor in Boston, who first introduced me to Chiropractic, to ask for his advice. He told me to contact his mentor Dr. Larry

Webster who was considered the grandfather of pregnancy and pediatric Chiropractic. Dr. Webster practiced in Atlanta.

Dr. Webster told me he knew exactly what to do to help Paula, but his office was too far away for us to drive to every week. He referred us to a local DC who had been trained in the Logan Basic Chiropractic technique. When this chiropractor started adjusting Paula, her contractions immediately lessened. Over the next few weeks, the frequency of her contractions decreased and eventually began to subside to the point where she was able to return to work.

Paula continued under his care throughout her pregnancy, and at forty weeks delivered a healthy baby boy. Both Paula and our son were so healthy that they were released by the hospital eighteen hours later.

We decided that the best way to thank Dr. Webster for his referral was to have him adjust our son. Seven days after our son was born, Dr. Webster gave him his first Chiropractic adjustment. Dr. Webster became one of my mentors throughout Chiropractic school and was influential in helping me open my first Chiropractic practice.

Paula and I have since delivered three more children at home, without any complications. In addition, I've been able to help pregnant women, newborns, and children throughout my Chiropractic career.

This personal experience taught our entire family to trust the inborn wisdom of the body and its ability to function better when it is free of nerve interference.

Paul Blumsack, DC
Blumsack Family Chiropractic
3770 Due West Rd., Suite 200
Marietta, GA 30064
770-362-6430
www.blumsackfamilychiropractic.com
Live Better ... Live Longer

"While other professions are concerned with changing the environment to suit the weak-ened body, Chiropractic is concerned with strengthening the body to suit the environment."

B. J. Palmer, DC

SECTION TWO

Infants
(Colic, Breast-feeding)

"The only way to be truly satisfied is to do what you believe is great work. And the only way to do great work is to love what you do."

Steve Jobs

From Breech to Breast-feeding

Dr. Alisha Davis

I met Dr. Davis in the beginning of my third trimester, when I was having intense back pain and could hardly walk at the end of a long day. Within a matter of a few adjustments, she had me not only walking but back to exercising and enjoying an energetic, happy pregnancy.

Near the end of my pregnancy, there was concern from my provider that the baby was breech. After a few gentle adjustments, the baby turned to the vertex position. Three days before my due date, my water broke and the baby had turned to a posterior position—not conducive for that fast, easy labor for which I was hoping.

I visited Dr. Davis that day, still not having contractions, and told her I needed that baby to turn to anterior and be in the best possible position for labor. Within a few minutes of her adjustment, we both felt the baby turn back around into an anterior position. The next morning, after a four-hour labor with only about fifteen minutes of pushing, I gave birth to a perfectly positioned nine-pound, twelve-ounce baby girl!

Dr. Davis called me the next day and I told her about my great birth experience. She asked how nursing was going. I thought to myself "How could this miracle worker of a person possibly help me with what I was experiencing with breast-feeding?" I told her the baby had a strong suck but was latching just to the end of my nipple and would not open her mouth very wide. (This was my third baby, and my other two had breast-fed for two years; but I was not sure if I could tolerate this agony for any length of time.) After only the first day, I was already very sore and had bleeding nipples.

Dr. Davis said, "Oh, let's get you in here and we'll get her to open her mouth wide."

My mom, who is a lactation specialist for a hospital in Maryland, was in town for the birth and had already tried every technique she knew to get Maeve to latch on better. She said she had never heard of Chiropractic for breast-feeding problems and was curious to see how it could help.

Maeve was just over 24 hours old when she had her first appointment with Dr. Davis. When we saw Dr. Davis at her office, we were nursing in the side-lying position. Maeve was sucking away with a tightly clenched jaw and I was in much pain. Lying on my side was the only position in which Maeve seemed to relax her jaw—a bit. She seemed to have a lot of tension in her head and didn't like it when I touched it too much or supported her neck.

Dr. Davis could immediately see the issue. Within only a few seconds of Dr. Davis adjusting her neck and performing gentle cranial work, Maeve's breathing changed completely. She took a deep breath, relaxed her jaw, and let her latch become much wider and took more of the breast into her mouth. It was the first time since she was born that both of us were relaxed while she was at breast.

My mother and I were both in awe. After I finished nursing, Dr. Davis did a few more adjustments on Maeve and we were off for our first day of more relaxed nursing. As days went by, Maeve would tighten up again, which is how I knew it was time for another adjustment. We initially saw Dr. Davis two or three days a week; then eventually just once a week for tune-ups. Without Dr. Davis's help, I'm not sure breast-feeding would have lasted very long.

I am a labor and delivery nurse and have recommended Dr. Davis to every woman I know who has back pain, fetal-positioning issues, or breast-feeding problems. Chiropractic, and especially my chiropractor, are amazing!

Alisha Davis, DC, DACCP
Davis Family Chiropractic, PLLC
7901 Strickland Road, Ste. 104
Raleigh, NC 27615
919-615-2257
www.davischironc.com
adavisdc@yahoo.com

Baby Seth

Dr. Amber Bush

Colic is one of those baby ailments that can drive a parent crazy and interrupt bonding due to exhaustion and lack of sleep for both the baby and the mother. When Megan walked into my office, carrying a crying infant, I could see the strain on her face. She had not slept, she was exhausted, and she had tried everything she could think of to appease her three-week-old baby boy. Nothing was working and no one was sleeping.

Seth was her second child. He was nothing like her first-born, who had slept well, was a happy baby, and all-in-all an "easy" baby.

Seth's birth was fairly uneventful; six hours of labor with no noted difficulties. He was breast-fed and had been doing well, eating every two hours like clockwork. He had no history of falling off the bed or any other injuries. He generally didn't sleep longer than two hours and had only one four-hour sleep since birth. Mom reported that he was fussy all the time and "hard to please." He was very gassy and had not had a bowel movement in ten days.

Following my evaluation, it was determined that Seth had subluxations in three areas of his spine: levels C2, T2, and L1. With use of gentle Chiropractic care, adjustments were made to T2 and L1, wanting to concentrate on his sympathetic nervous system. There was a general calm about Seth during his adjustment.

After Seth's first adjustment, Mom said his crying fits decreased some, and he slept three to four hours at a time twice a day for two days; and he moved his bowels the second day. He was rechecked two days after his first adjustment. On his third adjustment, Mom reported that he had been much better after the second adjustment, until three days later when he reverted to being fussier. She reported his bowel movements as normal.

I adjusted Seth five times. On his fifth re-check, no adjustment was needed. His spine was in alignment and his behavior was much improved. You could see on Mom's face that she was experiencing a sense of peace. I continued to check Seth monthly for an additional two months. Only one adjustment was given during that time, and then the family moved away.

Following her third pregnancy, I had the chance to treat Seth's mother again. She reported that he had continued to do well after his Chiropractic care. She was so grateful and recognized the value of checking children early on. Having had such a great experience with Seth, she brought her new baby in to be checked.

It is such an honor to be a part of a new child's life, knowing that Chiropractic can always make a positive difference.

Amber Bush, DC
Back to Balance Chiropractic
197 West Cherry Avenue
Porterville CA, 93257
559-783-2225
www.BacktoBalanceChiro.net

From Gastric Tube
to Eating in Four Months!

Dr. Bill Lawler

When I first met Finley, she was a tiny, five-month-old with multiple challenges. She was born twelve weeks early, and her two major difficulties were: At three months, she had transitioned from a fairly common premature-baby's nasogastric tube to a surgically installed gastric tube. Although her twin was able to eat normally after a few weeks, because of a semi-paralyzed mouth, Finley had not been able to eat anything orally. Therefore, she received all food via a gastric tube.

Her other major challenge was *hypertonia*, which is when the muscle tone is too high or rigid. Finley was not able to hold her head up on her own and often arched her back. She appeared uncomfortable most of the time, and also had a *torticollis* or a stiff neck.

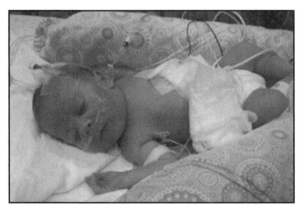

Her parents had taken her to multiple specialists, from pediatricians, rehabilitation therapists, etc. They had done multiple tests to see how to help Finley, but little to nothing was helping. While her twin, Tatum, was doing fairly well—bothered with some reflux and general fussiness—Finley was clearly struggling and not thriving.

Her parents brought Finley in, hoping that Chiropractic could do something to help their daughter who just wasn't coping very well with life.

Finley had multiple strikes against her, but using gentle cranio-sacral treatment (stimulating her skull and tailbone with light touch), what many might consider miracles occurred:

- After her first visit, she held up her head on her own for the first time ever.
- After her second visit, she yawned for the first time ever with a mostly balanced mouth.
- In the second week, she started to smile evenly.
- After a month, she started to suck on a pacifier
- Within two months, she was ready for a "swallow study."
- Within four months, she was feeding from a bottle and not a gastric tube.
- At six months, the gastric tube was totally removed.
- At eight months, she finally started to give her twin a run for her money

Finley's parents were amazed as they noticed more progress in her overall state after the first and second visits. They became emotional as they explained that this was an answer to their prayers. Dad was already thinking about becoming a chiropractor, so he could pay it forward to other infants like his daughter.

The magic of Chiropractic is shown from the tiniest of bodies. Finley just needed help to awaken the amazing intelligence inside her body that knew how to smile; open her mouth; suck; swallow; normalize muscle tone; and, in short, help her thrive. Additionally, her twin, Tatum, stopped having any fussiness, reflux, and sleeping difficulties after only a few gentle treatments as well.

Finley and Tatum are on their way to normal, amazing lives because their parents brought them to a pediatric chiropractor who removed interferences to their nervous systems and allowed their little bodies to do the rest.

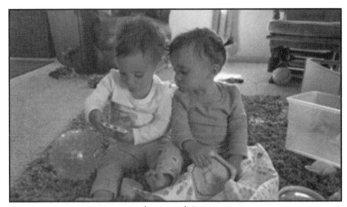

Finley and Tatum

When the body's healing powers are uncovered, miracles happen. After all, science has shown that the human body is self-developing, self-maintaining, and self-healing—provided there is no interference.

Bill Lawler, DC
Serving children and families for over 30 years
100 W. Canyon Crest Road, Suite 2
Alpine, UT 84004
801-492-0206
www.mychiro4kids.com

"The doctor of the future will give no medicine but will interest his patients in the care of the human frame, in diet and in the cause and prevention of disease."

THOMAS EDISON

A Grandmother's Plea

Dr. Birger Baastrup

About twenty years ago, I was travelling home to see my family in Denmark. My young son, who had a challenging birth a few years earlier, was accompanying us.

We had hoped for a home birth but ended up in the hospital. Labor proceeded very slowly, and eventually was not going where it should. The little tyke had turned around in the womb, which made his entry into this world even more difficult. But finally he was born, a perfect bundle of love.

We had some early challenges with him being fussy and crying frequently. None of us slept well for the first several months. I remember reading a study on colic and Chiropractic care (http://www.ncbi.nlm.nih.gov/pubmed/20937431) during that time period, which prompted me to have my son examined. Sure enough, he had a subluxation as a result of his birth and once corrected, he was great.

Back to our Denmark trip … we were visiting with relatives at my family's summerhouse grounds. My aunt started telling me about her newborn grandson. Evidently, my cousin's son had been colicky for a while and nothing they tried was giving him any relief.

Those of you who have experienced caring for a colicky child know how difficult it is to go through weeks and months of caring for someone you so dearly love and not being able to make them comfortable. You begin to feel sleep-deprived, totally drained, and frustrated at your inability to help the child, to the point where hopelessness often results.

Knowing what we had gone through with our son, my aunt asked if I might be able to help her grandson. I chatted with my cousins about their baby, and determined that it would be worth checking his spine. During a brief examination, I determined that the first vertebra in his neck (called the *atlas*) was out of alignment (*subluxated*). I proceeded to make the correction, and adjusted his C1 vertebra very gently.

After only one adjustment, his temperament and behavior completely turned. Irritation was removed and function was restored to his fragile nervous system. With happy baby, came the happy parents, and the very happy grandmother. The correction of that subluxation unified the family. And still to this day, my aunt raves about that adjustment.

The wonderful thing about adjusting babies is that they usually respond quickly, especially when they are checked and corrected early, which is why I suggest that all babies be checked for subluxation soon after birth, whether or not they have visible symptoms.

A healthy spine and nervous system are primordial to living a healthy life from birth.

Birger Baastrup, DC
800 Glacier Avenue
Juneau, AK 99801
907-463-5255

Baby Maria

Dr. Casey Sinclair

Maria was born full term at thirty-nine weeks and one day—a natural birth without any medication. Coming into this world, she was floppy and blue. It took four minutes for the medical team to reanimate her—to bring her back to life.

She was soon transferred to Toronto Sick Children's Hospital and spent the first three weeks of her life in the NICU. For thirteen of those days, she was on a ventilator. She was then transferred to general care for the next twenty-seven days. Yes, her first forty-eight days were spent in the hospital.

During her first week at home, I began visiting and adjusting Maria until she was ready to come into the clinic. Maria was adjusted on a frequency of two to three times per week. In addition, I performed ten minutes of neurological stimulation. Chiropractors focus on the nervous system. With the knowledge that every stimulus sends signals to the brain, it was important for Maria to have this brain stimulation to encourage as much development as possible. While most children will respond with a soft touch, activator, or manual adjustment, Maria needed more.

She initially experienced a lot of stress and her hands were always tightly clenched in a fist. They were clenched so tightly that it was nearly impossible to open her hand and spread her fingers. The rigid tone of her legs made it incredibly difficult for her mother to even change Maria's diapers.

With each adjustment, Maria's stress reduced and she became more relaxed; finally no longer making fists. Her eyes started to open more often. Simple tasks, like changing her diapers, became much easier for her mother. The only time Maria is vocal with sounds is during her adjustments, which is no surprise because this is when she is her most alert. She continues to improve and is showing us the body's unequivocal ability to heal.

Due to Maria's considerably lowered immune system, her Chiropractic care is critical to help reducing her chances of getting a simple cold or the flu, which for Maria could be life-threatening.

With children, there are always two stories; one about the child, and one about the parents. After Maria was born, her mother was experiencing panic attacks and generalized pain throughout her body. Bianca started getting adjusted regularly and, as a result, has been able to deal with her stress and is now pain-free.

Now that Bianca has experienced the benefits of Chiropractic care and has seen the benefits for Maria, she has also started bringing her three-year-old daughter, Melissa, in for care.

During a recent visit, Bianca said, "Thanks a lot, Dr. Casey and the Streetsville Chiropractic staff for being so great to us! I really believe that Maria will thank you by herself in the future. GOD bless you and all your family."

Casey Sinclair, DC
Streetsville Chiropractic
905-826-0900
www.streetsvillechiropractic.com
dr.casey@streetsvillechiropractic.com

Baby Karrington

Dr. Alisha Davis

My passion has always been to work with kids, which is why our practice focuses on pediatrics. Baby Karrington came into our office with her mother when she was only two months old. Her story is not much different than other babies that we see in the office, but this sweet, little girl has touched my heart.

Mom stated that she had a very stressful pregnancy and was hospitalized due to some medical conditions. Karrington's birth was very traumatic and she was delivered by a C-section and had to have the assistance of a vacuum delivery during the C-section!!! For her first two months of life, Karrington cried nonstop and Mom was unable to console her. Mom stated that she was not able to even leave the house because Karrington would not stop screaming. On average, Mom said she would cry for at least ten hours a day.

After taking Karrington multiple times to her pediatrician, she was started on reflux medications and encouraged to try every different formula on the market. Someone mentioned Chiropractic care … Mom's thoughts were that she would try anything to make her daughter better.

A chiropractor Mom knew from her hometown, who specialized in pediatrics, gave her our practice information. Karrington was seen for several weeks; and one week she came in every day for adjustments to improve the condition of the function of her nervous system.

Finally, Mom could see the light at the end of the tunnel!!! And, over the last week, Baby Karrington had almost a whole week of being a happy baby and only fussing for "normal" baby things, like a wet diaper, being sleepy, or hungry!!

What I love about this family is that the grandmother has even brought Karrington in for her adjustments when Mom has been unable to. They are committed to keeping Karrington on her recommended care plan. I remember the grandmother telling me, with tears in her eyes, that she finally got to see her granddaughter smile for the first time.

Mom has told everyone, "If your infant has any issues, take them immediately to Dr. Davis! I will never stop praising her name!!"

Children live their lives through their nervous system, and when stress impacts the nervous system, a child cannot grow, develop, or thrive. Stress on the nervous system impacts each of us differently, and for Karrington it was causing her to constantly cry out in pain. Removing the subluxations from her nervous system is allowing her to live life to her optimal potential!! When she comes in each week for her spinal checkup, you can see the light and sparkle in her eyes that she had been missing.

Chiropractic helped turn her power on!!

Alisha Davis, DC, DACCP
Davis Family Chiropractic, PLLC
7901 Strickland Road, Ste. 104
Raleigh, NC 27615
919-615-2257
www.davischironc.com
adavisdc@yahoo.com

Stella's Story

Dr. Crystal A. Galvan

From my own personal experience, I know the immense effect Chiropractic has on children, and I am compelled to share my vision with the world. As a child of Chiropractic, I saw many children come through my dad's office and have profound healing; so I knew it was possible, but I hadn't experienced it in my own practice yet. Then, Stella arrived!

Her mother brought her in to see me as a last resort, having gone the conventional route with no results. She was frustrated at having what she thought was no other option. Out of desperation, she did this without the consent of her husband. Stella was born by Cesarean section eight months prior and was diagnosed with Torticollis, caused by contraction of the right sterno-cleido mastoid (SCM) muscle at birth. Her mother reported that Stella was not able to turn her head to the left. She had a previous history of eye tearing, but no other major health concerns. After visiting with her primary care doctor and hearing about the invasive treatment options that were available, including surgery, she came to me for help.

After a thorough examination of Stella, I discovered a subluxated first cervical vertebra (called the atlas), as well as a posterior sacral base (bone at bottom of spine that forms part of the pelvis). Stella's head had a significant right-head tilt, especially noticeable when looking at her from the front, with a slight chin rotation to the left. There was also visual confirmation of the sacral misalignment. Neurological and orthopedic tests were all within normal limits. She JUST could not turn her head to the left!

This may sound simple to some; however, I realized that

this was a complex case and I was very excited to help this baby girl with potentially lifelong benefits. Initially, we started care with minimal frequency and low-force adjustments of Stella's subluxated spinal segments. She responded with improved sleep and some improvement in range of motion.

I treated her eight times over the next eight months using the Activator Method, with the same results. I knew that her mother was having a hard time keeping the secret of her Chiropractic care from her husband and needed to get some drastic results. So, on her last visit, my intuition told me that she needed a little bit more movement in the cervical spine. I performed a high-velocity low-force manual adjustment, with minimal rotation, that produced multiple audible releases; the sounds often heard when a joint moves during an adjustment.

Mom and Stella were a bit surprised by the "new" adjustment, but then the BIG surprise came when Stella turned her head to the left for the first time in her life. She was most definitely surprised at her newfound ability to look over her shoulder! I will always remember her face and the expression of surprise. Every year at Christmas I get my favorite card from one of my most memorable patients, Stella!

My vision for Chiropractic is that every child and adult will commit to improving their quality of life with lifelong care of their body's nervous system by getting regular Chiropractic adjustments.

Crystal A. Galvan, DC
310 Pine Ave. Suite B
Goleta, CA 93117
805-687-8900
www.dr-cc.com

From Starving to Well-Fed

Dr. Dina Sgambati

Last February, a new mom and her two-week-old son came to the office with latching difficulties. Mom was at her wits' end and said they had gotten off to a rough start with breast-feeding. Each attempt would consist of this little guy desperately trying to latch for over an hour. Then she would give up, resign herself to pumping, and feed him with a syringe due to worries about nipple confusion. (Eventually she switched to a bottle after seeking the advice of her pediatrician.)

On the rare occasion when a successful latch occurred, it would never last long. He would quickly lose the latch, leaving his mother in tears of frustration and her newborn screaming from hunger.

Mom was miserable, sleep-deprived, and feeling very unsuccessful as a mother. She met with a lactation consultant. She was told that her nipples were flat, making it difficult for her son to get a strong latch. The consultant provided techniques to draw her nipples out a bit more, but the results were marginal.

That's when her husband said, "Let's take him to Dr. Sgambati for an adjustment." Interestingly, her husband's father was a chiropractor. Although his dad had suddenly passed away when her husband was only ten years old, the principles of Chiropractic had made a lasting impression on him.

Not only had she received prenatal Chiropractic care upon his recommendation, but now she would be bringing in her newborn son for his first adjustment as well!

A Chiropractic evaluation for a newborn, to assess any stresses and strains from the birth process, was not a concept she had grown up with, but she trusted her husband enough to know it was a good decision.

During the examination, I was able to assess the muscle tone and motion of each spinal segment with my pinky finger while his mother held him comfortably in her arms. A technique referred to as "surrogate muscle testing" assisted me in the detection of any subluxations. I adjusted the top bone in his neck on the left, as well as a few segments in the thoracic spine using an adjusting tool that feels like a slight vibration to the baby.

After the appointment, they went home and immediately sat down to give breast-feeding a try. She said she remembers crying and pleading with the hope that it would work. She was willing to try for just one more day because she truly felt like she was losing it.

To her amazement, her son latched on immediately. She couldn't believe it! This had never happened before! He breast-fed for almost an hour the first time, and alternated easily from one breast to the other. She was crying hysterically and declared him the "breast-feeding champion"! She maintains that from the time of that first adjustment they never had latch-related issues again.

She has said it many times, and will say it again and again, that her son's Chiropractic adjustment saved her breast-feeding career.

Dr. Sgambati, a prenatal chiropractor and mother of two, has pursued advanced training to establish a maternity specialty. She is an active member of the American Pregnancy Association, the International Chiropractic Pediatric Association, and is Webster Technique certified. A contributing writer for many publications, including the *North Jersey Expectant Mother's Guide*, *Hoboken Digest* and *Hoboken Family Alliance Newsletter*; Dr. Sgambati was also honored to participate in the award-winning documentary Orgasmic Birth alongside many world-renowned birth experts.

Dina Sgambati, DC
Priority Chiropractic
51 Newark St., Suite 205
Hoboken, NJ 07030
201-533-1077
www.prioritychironj.com

Revived Hope

Dr. David DeMoulin

I always smile when I hear a patient say the phrase "Chiropractic can help with that?" That statement of disbelief makes me smile because I love seeing patients' eyes open to the healing power that exists inside their body.

One day, a grandmother was telling me her worries about her newborn grandson. He had torticollis; he couldn't tilt his head left, he could barely hold his head center. He was colicky and having major breast-feeding issues. The pediatrician prescribed physical therapy and changes were slow. The biggest concern this grandmother had was that her daughter was going to have to stop breast-feeding her newborn because he would only nurse on one side and he was not gaining weight.

I told her, "Bring him in. We need to check for a neurological cause. If there is one, we can help."

I could tell she was about to use the phrase I love to hear. She was skeptical. She had been told it was a "muscular" problem and that the baby was positioned awkwardly in the womb to cause the condition. She didn't see how the nervous system could be involved. After a brief conversation about the potential effects birth trauma can have on a newborn's spine, especially a birth with heavy medical intervention, she was onboard—at least for a consultation and exam.

A few days later, this little baby arrived with his mother, and of course, Grandma in tow. His head was tilted to the right and his chin pointed at the ceiling. It was a sad sight, seeing a new mom visibly stressed and a helpless baby just wanting a chance for a normal start in life.

The baby's mom told me the troubles her little guy was having and how she had developed a depressive loss of hope.

The baby would only nurse for two minutes at a time and only on one side. I desperately wanted to revive a sense of hope in this mom.

After a short, yet thorough, examination, it was conclusive that this baby had a major misalignment in his neck. This was the light I was looking for. His vertebra had slid out of proper position and had caused serious neurologic compromise.

After discussing the findings with Mom, I was ready to restore life to this child and hope to his mother. Even though trust had been established, Mom was still apprehensive. Using the right pressure in the right direction on his tiny bone, I gave her son his first Chiropractic adjustment. After ten seconds, he held his head up, dead center.

Mother and son returned two days later, and Mom reported Baby was getting full feedings at five minutes on both sides. He had gained almost six ounces in those two days. She was ecstatic.

After two additional visits, the baby's torticollis was completely resolved. He was gaining weight and finally sleeping more than a few hours at a time.

It goes to show, you can never put Chiropractic in a box. One adjusted baby can give an entire family their lives back.

David DeMoulin, DC
DeMoulin Family Chiropractic
Greater Chicago, Illinois
www.demoulinchiro.com

The Importance of
Proper Alignment for Breast-feeding

Dr. Laura T. Brayton

Holly is the absolute pride and joy of her parents, Tiffany and Fred, who went through countless fertility treatments in order to conceive their healthy baby girl. Holly's mama received her first Chiropractic adjustments at the end of her pregnancy due to breech positioning. However, Holly did not turn head down into the vertex position; therefore, she entered the world via Caesarean section on July 7, 2015.

Holly was only five weeks old when her mother brought her in for Chiropractic care. From the very beginning, Tiffany noticed that Holly favored looking in one direction and did not appear to have full range of motion in her neck. And there were challenges with nursing. Holly would frequently pull off the nipple and cry in frustration; as well as not get enough milk during the feedings.

Tiffany had undertaken the arduous task of exclusively pumping and supplementing the pumped breast milk with some formula. As an educated mama, Tiffany was committed to providing breast milk for her baby; however, her entire life revolved around pumping and feeding and she was exhausted.

When Tiffany came into the office after the birth to get her spine checked for misalignments (*subluxations*), she shared with me her nursing challenges. I immediately suggested she bring in her baby to also get checked for subluxations due to potential strain from in-utero positioning and from the surgical birth. Tiffany agreed to give it a try after I explained the gentleness of a newborn adjustment and also the effectiveness for removing interference to the nervous system, allowing the body to function at an optimal level.

A couple days later, little Holly lay on a pillow in my office while I calmly felt the alignment at the top of her neck as well as her jaw and cranial bones. Once I detected the subtle misalignments that could contribute to latching issues, my skilled fingers delicately went to work to correct the positions. When I finished Holly's adjustment, I handed her over to her mama and suggested that she attempt to nurse when she got home from the appointment. Tiffany lifted an eyebrow with some doubt, but agreed she would give it a try.

This is the email I received the next day:

> Hi Dr. Brayton,
> I wanted to tell you ... Holly latched on after I got home and took your advice to try breast-feeding after you had adjusted her! Thank you so much for working your magic!
> Tiffany

I have adjusted Holly two other times in the past few weeks to help maintain her correct alignment; yet she has not had any other issues with her latch since the first adjustment. I am honored to be able to serve the mothers and babies in my practice at such a deep, intimate level.

Laura T. Brayton, DC, CACCP
Hoboken Chiropractic + Wellness, Inc.
50 Harrison St., Suite 316
Hoboken, NJ 07030
201-792-3544
www.HobokenChiro.com

A Happy Mother

Dr. Laura Stone

I want to tell you the amazing story of how Chiropractic care changed the life of my baby boy, Henry.

Unfortunately, Henry, my third child, was born with a broken clavicle, a consequence of a rigorous birthing process. As a nurse, I knew this was a fairly common occurrence; however, I also questioned the amount of traumatic stress his little body might have suffered in-utero and the physical stress he might have been under during my entire pregnancy.

Thus, my husband and I set up his initial appointment with our family chiropractor, Dr. Laura Stone. Before beginning Chiropractic care, Henry was on three different medications for acid reflux and colic. Immediately after his first gentle adjustment, my husband and I started noticing positive changes in our precious baby boy. His reflux became nonexistent and he was no longer on any prescribed medications. He was happier and more vocal than our two other children were at that stage.

I continue to tell people that with Chiropractic care, Henry is just more active. Specifically, he babbles and communicates vocally throughout the entire day, at five months young. Dr. Laura emphasizes that Chiropractic care can be the key to a happy and healthy baby. It is TRUE! Henry is, indeed, a happy baby!

In addition to the increased vocalizations, Henry is also exceeding all of his developmental milestones for his age. We have witnessed Henry rolling in both directions and almost sitting up on his own. He is also able to place equal body weight on both legs and is showing signs that he wants to crawl. If I see an occasional ear tug and detect a slight fever, we take Henry to get adjusted. Dr. Laura uses a heat-detecting instrument to find the areas of the spine that need to be worked on and she adjusts Henry accordingly. His body works more effectively at fighting off illness quicker. It's AMAZING!

Chiropractic care is the key to all of these wonderful and healthy changes in Henry, and for that we are very thankful. I only regret not knowing how important and beneficial Chiropractic care is to infants, toddlers, and children when first becoming a parent. Perhaps there could have been some avoidable illnesses and fewer prescriptions for my first two.

I continue to be excited to share with others the numerous benefits Chiropractic care has for all stages of life.

(written by Courtney, Henry's mother)

Laura Stone, DC, MS
Family First Chiropractic Center
510 State Ave., Suite #3
Hampton, IL 61256
309-751-9790
Family1stchiropractic.com

Wondering, Watching, and Waiting

Dr. Laura Gravelle

Our adventure during the month of July 2013 was just that, a venture into unknown and uncharted territory.

When you have a baby in the Neonatal Intensive Care Unit (NICU) your days become all consumed with wondering, watching, and waiting. You wonder: What are the doctors thinking? What will they do next? How is your baby doing?

You watch … as the tubes and needles go in and out of that fragile, little human; as all of the doctors and specialists and nurses come and going.

You wait. You wait. And you wait some more. Your mind wonders about all sorts of what-ifs. You do your best to stay positive as the test results come back; you wait for your baby to grow, and you wait to go home.

There were days that were very scary, very calm, very "going through the motions," and very emotional. There were days when I talked a lot and others when I didn't.

When you are in the center of a spiral that seems to spin and spin and spin, you just want it to stop … if even just for a minute.

Then, one day, it did stop. The day I will always remember is when the NICU neonatologist said, "All of Lucy's problems seem to be going away." That was a wonderful, brilliant day.

I know the intelligence that made her body is that which is now supporting all healing, growth, and repair. The day after we had Lucy's spine checked and adjusted by my colleague and friend Dr. Peter Amlinger, her body chemistry began to normalize … all of her chemistry that was out of balance began to get to normal. (Though I am a chiropractor, I needed someone outside of my emotional connection to check her. I needed his expertise.)

Gases that were high came down; gases that were low came up. Her Ph (acid-base balance) that was low, came up; her breathing normalized; and markers in her blood were gone.

Dr. Amlinger adjusted Lucy's upper cervical spine and occiput (skull). He believes that her speedy entrance into this world (fifteen minutes from 6 cm to 10 cm dilation and immediate birth) was a severe shock to her fragile nervous system.

I knew that 100 percent connection and support of all body functions through the nervous system is necessary; and, when it is not present, the body is unable to adapt as it is designed to. After the adjustment, we waited for Lucy to adapt to this new earthly environment with hope and expectation … then we watched and waited for all the MDs to be amazed, for test results to come back clear, for her body to heal, for time to be on our side … to go home.

Chiropractic care absolutely changed the course of her healing and our stay in the hospital. The day all the tubes came out was the day she began to gain weight. We were able to bring Lucy home.

We are so very thankful for the care of the NICU team, for their compassion, knowledge, and expertise. We are so thankful for their medical expertise. I know in my heart, that the combination of Western allopathic care, Chiropractic, and other energetic healing practices we employed to support our baby helped make her well, the way she was designed to be— the way all babies are designed to be.

I continue to check to see how Lucy holds her adjustments. She is thriving (not just surviving), growing, and glowing. We wonder, watch, and wait to see how this little medical mystery continues to exemplify the Chiropractic principle: "The power that made the body is the power that heals."

Live your best life, get adjusted!

Laura Gravelle, DC
Gravelle Family Chiropractic and Wellness Centre
350 Oxford Street West, Suite 202
London, Ontario
519-433-9222
www.chirolaura.com and www.adjustyourpractice.ca
https://twitter.com/ChiroLauraG
Drlauragravelle.blogspot.ca

Baby Tatum

Dr. Liz Homan

Baby Tatum came in when she was six weeks old, after having extreme fussiness since she was two weeks old. This was hard for mom, because she could tell that her baby was in pain, but she didn't know how to help her. Mom decided to try Chiropractic for Tatum after seeing positive results in her older daughter for similar issues when she was a baby.

Tatum's fussiness was typically worse in the morning and evening, and while nursing. When nursing, she would thrash around in pain, which made it difficult for her to get a full feeding. This was very difficult on mom, too, who at times, questioned if she would be able to continue breast-feeding her new baby. Tatum would cry most nights from 10:00 p.m. until midnight, which for any parent can be draining.

While talking with mom, it was determined that there likely had been severe stress put on Tatum's spine during the birth process. Labor had lasted seven hours, requiring Mom to push twelve times. An evaluation of Tatum's spine was completed and reduced motion was found when she turned her head. This could cause pain while breast-feeding and result in thrashing. It was found that when light pressure was applied over her low back, Tatum would squirm away to try to stop it from happening. This area of the spine is responsible for supplying the digestive system, and irritation could cause fussiness when being laid down on her back for sleep.

Once the areas of involvement were determined, a light, specific adjustment was performed in order to restore proper function. I explained to Mom that the pressure of the adjustment would be about the same as what you would use to check the ripeness of a tomato and would result in the realignment of the bones so the body could heal. A few hours after the adjust-ment, mom shared that while nursing, there was no thrashing. And, after that feeding, Tatum took a nap in her crib and fell asleep on her own, instead of crying for at least thirty minutes before falling asleep.

On their following visit, Baby Tatum looked happy and Mom was excited to announce that there had only been three episodes of thrashing while feeding the entire weekend, when previously it was every time.

Tatum has continued to sleep well. In the weeks following the initial visit, Mom would occasionally report that Tatum was getting fussy with feedings, but after a specific adjustment, the feedings would improve substantially. Overall, Tatum was much more relaxed during the day, which means that Mom was also more relaxed.

At four months old, Tatum is able to continue nursing with comfort, and is doing beautifully. She continues to get checked for subluxations, and when necessary receives specific Chiropractic spinal adjustments to make sure that her nervous system and entire body are working properly and helping her become a healthy, happy kid!

Liz Homan, DC
Infinite Life Chiropractic Center
5870 Zarley Street, Suite B
New Albany, Ohio 43054
614-289-8728
www.InfiniteLifeChiro.com
www.facebook.com/InfiniteLifeChiropractic

Jasper's Journey

Dr. Preston Pierce

When I first set eyes on Jasper, he was only four months old and his parents knew absolutely nothing about Chiropractic care. Thankfully, a close friend understood enough to recommend that they bring the baby in to see me. I noticed right away that about 80 percent of little Jasper's body was covered in a painful, bumpy red rash—similar to a diaper rash, but not confined to his diaper area. It was equally obvious that he was struggling with the amount of mucous his body was producing throughout his respiratory system. He had been consistently sick since birth and his weakened immune system was not able to fight effectively. The poor guy was not a happy dude. It was heart-wrenching to see.

Jasper's mom informed me that in addition to the obvious infection and dermatitis, he had also been diagnosed with asthma, reflux, and colic. His digestion, she said, was a mess, and Jasper was constipated most of the time. Almost immediately after birth, Jasper's pediatrician prescribed the following: round after round of antibiotics, steroid cream, Zantac, and Prilosec! I was in shock, to say the least.

During further consultation, I learned there had been complications, both during pregnancy and during birth. Not surprisingly, while examining the infant through motion and static palpation, I found restrictions (subluxations) of the C0 (skull), C1 (neck), L3, L5 (low back) and S2 (pelvis).

True to my heart as a chiropractor, I decided that Jasper's course of treatment must include attention to the whole of his being—physical, mental/emotional, and biochemical. We scheduled him for routine adjustments of his nervous system, beginning with three times a week for three weeks, then weaning down slowly (two visits per week, one visit per week, etc.), as he progressed. I encouraged his family to give Jasper lots of attention, to touch him, and love on him.

I want to be clear on this next point: as a chiropractor, I am not licensed to take anyone off prescribed medications. HOWEVER, after bringing Jasper to see me, his parents immediately stopped giving Jasper the Prilosec and Zantac, while adding what I recommended: probiotics for his digestive system. As Jasper's age permitted, I encouraged his parents to feed him whole, raw, organic foods and to avoid sugars and processed items.

Children are resilient. They are born with a body, complete with its own natural ability to self-heal—we call it *innate intelligence*! So, when we removed the interference Jasper was

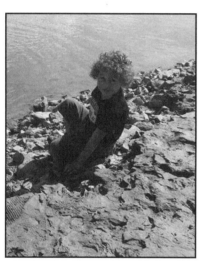

experiencing in his nervous system and his biochemistry, amazing things began to happen. His body took over and did what it does best ... it healed.

The first thing to change was Jasper's temperament. His colic subsided and smiles became commonplace. The reflux and constipation gradually became the exception rather than the rule. Eventually, his extreme skin condition also began to slowly clear up!

Years later, the question still haunts me: What if his parents were never told that Chiropractic could be much more than mere pain relief? Where would this little boy be today?

Preston Pierce, DC
Natural Touch Wellness Center
Kansas City and Overland Park, KS
913-284-2949
naturaltouchwc@gmail.com

Jacob's Story

Dr. Rebecca Lamarche

Nothing pulls at my heart more than seeing a mother at the end of her rope, desperately trying to get the right care for her child. That was the scenario I walked into when I met Amy and her son, Jacob.

Jacob was adorable. His bright-blue eyes shined up at me from his mother's lap. During our consultation, Amy told me how she had been talking with a friend who was a patient in our office. The friend was concerned that Jacob, who was now nine months old, was not crawling yet.

Jacob was Amy's second child, and she had noticed other differences between him and her older daughter. Jacob just didn't seem to be a happy baby. He didn't smile, laugh, or interact with her the way her first child did. Although she was well aware that every child is different, Amy felt something was not right. Many would call that "mother's intuition."

She brought Jacob to a chiropractor because she thought he might have something wrong with his hips or pelvis that made it painful for him to crawl, and possibly the discomfort was affecting his demeanor. As we talked more about Jacob's history, she revealed that he had suffered a few ear infections in his short life, and he was frequently sick.

Upon examination, I discovered areas of subluxation in Jacob's low back, pelvis, and cervical spine. I explained to Amy that subluxation could cause discomfort and limit Jacob's range of motion. I also explained how the brain communicates to the rest of the body via the spinal cord, and how nerves branch out, bringing energy to every cell, tissue, and organ. Having a subluxation disrupts optimal communication from the brain to body.

Amy looked amazed at hearing this newfound knowledge. "You know, he gets constipated a lot. Could that have anything to do with the subluxation you found in his low back?" Amy asked.

"Absolutely!" I answered. It's one of the highlights of my day to see a patient go from knowing Chiropractic can help with musculoskeletal issues to understanding how keeping the spine and nervous system healthy allows the whole body to function at an optimal level.

Jacob got his first adjustment that day. Over the next few weeks, as I kept adjusting him, his body was quickly healing from the inside out.

Amy first noticed Jacob was sleeping better and having bowel movements more frequently. As we continued care, Jacob went from sitting longer, to trying to get in a crawling stance, to actually making his first crawling movements. Amy reported that Jacob was interacting more with her, smiling, and overall had a happier demeanor. Her eyes welled up with happy tears when she explained how excited she was to have finally found the solution Jacob so desperately needed.

What a joy it is, as a chiropractor, to help a mother find a solution for her child and to help a child get the best possible start in life.

Rebecca Lamarche, DC
ReVive Health Centre
3420 Lacrosse Lane, Suite 100, Office 2
Naperville, IL 60564
630-637-3420
www.ReViveHealthCentre.com

From Pain to Function

Dr. Tim Wood and
Dr. Suzie Wood

Helping children live life closer to their potential for health, happiness, and impacting others is a rewarding part of being a family chiropractor. We hear so many stories of how lives are changed through Chiropractic. Science has shown that over 85 percent of the neurological change from an adjustment affects things that people cannot feel; so the patient's excited changes are only the tip of the iceberg!

One of my hockey mates explained that his newborn son seemed unhappy and wouldn't sleep. I offered to check him to see if there was nerve interference from misalignment in his spine. Here is a factual recollection from the child's mother:

"My son has been in Dr. Tim's care for six months. My husband and I brought him to the office when he was five weeks old. He was having difficulty sleeping. He would nap comfortably in his car seat and when he was in a reclined position, but anywhere else he would get fussy. Whenever he was in a prone position, he appeared to be in pain. He would cry, kick his legs, and curl his knees. We thought he had gastric problems and did our best to alleviate his symptoms.

"He was sleeping very little, maybe four or five hours a night and wasn't napping during the daytime. I've always been an advocate of Chiropractic care; so I was relieved to know that Tim worked on infants as well. We had our first consultation and Tim found Morgan's problem in one visit: a neck vertebra misalignment, which was likely the result of him being born by emergency C-section.

"After Morgan's first adjustment, he slept eight hours!! My husband and I felt like we were on vacation! Our son is now eight months old and hasn't been sick once, not even a cold!

We continue to have him checked and adjusted when necessary, especially since he's crawling. He continues to improve and is a very happy, active baby who loves to come to see his chiropractor every two weeks."

Tim Wood, DC and Suzie Wood, DC
Mission Family Chiropractic
#10 – 3818 Gordon Dr.
Kelowna, BC V1W 4V1
250-712-0900
www.missionchiropractic.ca
info@missionchiropractic.ca

Plagiocephaly

Dr. Erin Jones

When Jaylyn called to make an appointment for her son, Judah, I assumed we would be having a general wellness visit. I had cared for Jaylyn during her pregnancy and we had discussed the benefits of Chiropractic care for newborns. Judah was about four months old; so I was looking forward to meeting him and checking for any subluxations or misalignments that may have occurred during the birth process or since then.

It took me by surprise when I learned Jaylyn's main concern for Judah was the shape, or rather misshape, of his head. Judah had developed a flat right spot on the back of his head, as well as a bulge on the right side of his forehead. (This is a relatively common condition in babies called *plagiocephaly*, which can be caused by the position of the baby in-utero or sleeping on his back for an extended period of time.)

Jaylyn had also noticed Judah favored turning his head to the right and mainly used his right arm. Her concern was enough that she had consulted with Judah's pediatrician about his head shape. They were referred to a pediatrics plastics specialist whom they had an appointment with the following week. Typical medical treatment for plagiocephaly is helmet therapy, where the baby wears a helmet as long as five months. This usually costs thousands of dollars.

After examining Judah, I located upper cervical subluxations as well as cranial bone imbalances that needed to be addressed. The adjustment went well and Judah didn't mind too much when I found some sore spots.

I recommended that he get checked and adjusted when needed twice per week over the next five weeks and then we could re-evaluate. A baby's cranial bones are not fused yet and it is much easier to make changes the sooner they are addressed. From my experience working with children, I knew that Judah should respond quickly to Chiropractic adjustments. I had high hopes for his progress.

At their next appointment, Jaylyn was thrilled to report the noticeable difference on Judah's forehead. It had balanced out beautifully and the bulge on the right side was barely noticeable. This was encouraging enough to Judah's parents that they cancelled his appointment with the pediatric plastic specialist. After another adjustment, I demonstrated at-home exercises that mom and dad could do with Judah to facilitate his care. By the time the next visit rolled around, Judah had started to use his left arm and hand more often and the back of his head was beginning to show more balance.

The following week, Judah's head shape was looking nice and smooth; Mom was amazed! He was continuing to use his left hand equally with his right. We continued with his treatment plan so that the underlying issue and subluxation would be fully corrected. We then transitioned to a maintenance plan to support a healthy childhood.

Today Judah is a happy, healthy sixteen-month-old. His parents are still thrilled with the fast response of balancing his head shape through Chiropractic care, as well as the thousands of dollars potentially saved by choosing Chiropractic first!

Dr. Erin Jones is a Palmer College of Chiropractic graduate. She focuses on prenatal, pediatric, and family Chiropractic care in her clinic, Seasons of Health Chiropractic. Her passion is educating patients and the community on alternative health care and patient empowerment through Chiropractic, nutrition, and essential oils.

Erin Jones, DC
Seasons of Health Chiropractic
3201 S. Providence Rd., Suite 204
Columbia, MO 65203
573-214-2737
www.SeasonsofHealth.com
facebook.com/seasonsofhealthchiropractic

The Story of David

Dr. Doug Fryday

About thirty years ago, soon after I bought my practice, my assistant came into the adjusting room and said a horse and buggy just pulled up and an Amish family was coming into the office. I came out and greeted a mom and dad and a slew of kids ranging from a newborn, who was crying hysterically, to a young teen. There were seven in total, all dressed in the traditional Amish attire. They were here because of David, the newborn. He was a week old and hadn't stopped crying since he was born, said the mother.

With desperation in her voice, she asked, "Do you think you can help him?"

> **"You never know how far-reaching something you think, say or do today will affect the lives of millions tomorrow."**
>
> B. J. PALMER, DC

"Of course, I can!" I blurted, with a tremendous amount of silent skepticism in my head.

You see, as a newbie chiropractor, barely, in practice for three months, I was lacking experience, but I was strong on enthusiasm! After all, I had been trained at Palmer College of Chiropractic, the fountainhead, the Harvard of Chiropractic schools. This should be a piece of cake!

They brought David back to the adjusting room and I got the mother to lie down with him on her belly so that he would feel a secure. I examined his tiny spine for subluxations, in between his big screams and spasms that brought his knees to his chest. I found an atlas subluxation, the first bone in the spine that your head sits on. I suspected the birthing process was the cause, as the mom said he had been stuck in the birth canal for over three hours!

I gently and specifically adjusted his atlas. David immediately stopped screaming and melted into his mother's body! I quietly said thank you to the Creator and told the parents I would come out to their farm the next day to check up on "little" David. Almost thirty years later, I am looking after "big" David's family!

This first encounter with baby David was the start of a beautiful relationship with the Amish community.

I opened a satellite office closer to their community, to make it easier for them to travel to the office. Every second Wednesday, I travel to seven Amish farms and adjust families; three generations is not uncommon.

I feel privileged to serve these kind, gentle people who truly live a Chiropractic lifestyle. What I have observed over the years, is that the Amish children seem to be healthier than the children in my community. Amish children expose themselves every day to bugs by playing outside, and even run in the barnyard in bare feet. They drink raw cow's milk, favor natural food over processed food, and refuse to vaccinate. The adults rarely experience disorders like cancer and cardiovascular disease, and very rarely come down with colds or flu.

The Amish have a high level of physical activity due to the fact that they rely on "human power" and not machinery. They have a huge sense of family and community. Oftentimes there are three generations living on the same farm, and they always gather together for meals. They are very social, and visit with their neighbors most nights.

They love to joke and laugh, which is something I didn't expect—but I welcome every time. I am sure they have stress in their lives, but it's not like ours. They live in a "simple" world, where we live in a "pressure-cooker" world!

The biggest things I have learned from my Amish friends is to pull in the reins on this journey of life, live simple, move more, laugh often, and take time to connect with your community and the land. If you take the first step, you will always get to where you are going!

Thank you, David!

Dr. Doug Fryday is a wellness lifestyle expert who has been in practice in Saugeen Shores for thirty years. He specializes in brain-based Chiropractic, with a special interest in how stress affects the brain and ultimately your life.

Doug Fryday, DC
Optimize Family Chiropractic
625 Goderich St.
Port Elgin, ON Canada N0H 2C0
519-832-1515
www.optimizehealing.com

The Importance of Being Able to Nurse

Dr. Wendy N. Sanches

One Tuesday afternoon, an adorable newborn boy named Jonathan was brought into my office by his first-time mother. Jonathan was having difficulty nursing. Despite efforts under the evaluation and instruction of a Lactation Consultant (IBCLC), Jonathan and his mother had not been able to establish healthy nursing. The IBCLC referred them to my office over concern of a mechanical issue of the jaw or upper-cervical region of the spine, which had caused four-day-old Jonathan to lose about fifteen ounces since birth.

His mother stated that Jonathan was chomping down on her when he tried to nurse, causing her a lot of pain and discomfort.

He was unable to form a correct suction on the breast to force a letdown of milk, allowing him to gain the appropriate weight for proper development.

Because of these issues, mother and baby were unable to create a beneficial and enjoyable nursing bond essential in the first days of life.

When I asked Jonathan's mother about her pregnancy, she stated she had the typical first-trimester morning sickness but enjoyed pregnancy once the symptoms ended. She also acknowledged experiencing pubic symphysis pain (pain in the front of the pelvis) in the last couple months of her pregnancy. Jonathan was head down and ready to go when he was born at thirty-eight weeks and six days gestation.

His mother labored for eighteen hours and pushed for four hours. He was born at a birth center with a midwife and was welcomed into this world by being immediately placed on his mother's chest for warmth and love. He weighed eight pounds, twelve ounces and was twenty-one inches long. His mother stated that the pushing phase of her delivery was very challenging and she experienced a lot of pubic pain even after the delivery.

Upon visual evaluation of Jonathan, his head was tilted to the left, he had a right high ear, head rotation to the right, and a high left shoulder. Jonathan was also born with a left club foot. Cranial evaluation revealed a left parietal bulge, left temporal/parietal overlap, and a left parietal/frontal overlap, and he presented with a left sacral apex. These are all terms suggesting concerns with the position of his cranial bones and his sacrum. All other orthopedic and neurological evaluations were within normal limits.

I started by adjusting Jonathan's left C1 (atlas, first bone below the skull). Following this adjustment, he started to correct his head tilt and rotation back to the midline. Then I adjusted the left sacral apex. I performed some cranial adjustments to help the cranial bones to become "unstuck" and shift back to their correct position. I then adjusted his left Temporo Mandibular Joint (TMJ). After balancing the cranium, I then did some Craniosacral Therapy (CST) to balance the rhythm of the occiput and sacrum, in order to balance cerebral spinal fluid (CSF) pressure throughout the brain and spinal cord.

At the second visit two days later, Jonathan's mother reported that he was no longer chomping at her breast; however he was not suckling very well. At this visit, I found his left C1 and left sacrum still subluxated. I adjusted those segments, worked on his cranium, and adjusted his right TMJ. I also evaluated the palate and found that it was dropped on the left side.

After correcting all of these subluxations and correcting the Cranial Rhythmic Impulse (CRI, cranial bones correction) and CST, Jonathan began to nurse well and had gained three ounces by the time he came in for his next visit.

Jonathan is now thirteen months old. He has continued a nourishing nursing relationship and maintains a healthy weight. He still receives regular Chiropractic adjustments and recently he took his first steps, much to the delight of his mother. His infectious smile lights up my office. He is a very happy and healthy little boy.

Wendy N. Sanches, DC
Family Chiropractor
Empowered Life, PC
106 International Drive
Rincon, GA 31326
912-826-3482
912-655-3319 (Cell)
drwendysanches@gmail.com
www.EmpoweredLifeChiropractic.com

The Importance of
Proper Nerve Supply for Latching

Dr. Jeanne Engert Sandheinrich

A mother brought her eighteen-day-old infant in to see me because she heard that Chiropractic care might help with the baby latching during breast-feeding. Ellie was the third child in the family and her mother desperately wanted to breast-feed her baby like the other two.

Ellie had not latched well on the breast since birth. It was reported that the two days prior to her first visit, she was only able to feed at the breast one time because she was not getting enough milk and it was painful for her mother to continue. Ellie was not tilting her head back far enough to allow her mouth to open wide. She had a very shallow latch and short sucks. Her mother also noticed that Ellie favored turning her head to the right.

The mother and father were finger feeding her pumped breast milk to maintain the milk supply and get the baby good nutrients. So far, Ellie was gaining weight, but it was becoming a concern that she was not feeding at the breast properly.

During examination, it was determined that Ellie had a disorganized suck. She had subluxations in the sacrum, upper neck, base of the skull, and many cranial bones including the sphenoid, temporal, and maxilla. I explained to the mother that a subluxation is a misalignment in the spine that is not moving properly. When the spine is not moving properly, the nervous system cannot efficiently send the proper signals to the rest of the body. Adjustments at the upper neck and base of the skull would also balance the nervous system, specifically the vagus nerve, to allow the tongue and muscles in the throat to work effectively.

I performed a gentle adjustment to the spine and cranium,

with my fingers, giving as much pressure as I would put on a peach without bruising it. I explained to the mother that we needed to get the bones to move properly again in the skull so that Ellie could open her mouth and suck correctly.

The baby received the adjustment very well. She was sleeping through most of the treatment. After the adjustment, I asked the mother to attempt a feeding and come to the front desk when she was finished. Thirty minutes later, the mother came out of the adjustment room with the biggest smile on her face. With tears in her eyes, she exclaimed, "She fed perfectly and on both sides!"

They returned a week later and the mother reported that this beautiful baby girl was still feeding at the breast, but it was still a little painful and the latch seemed shallow. After the fourth treatment, she was no longer having pain while nursing and doing much better overall.

Chiropractic care was able to keep the breast-feeding relationship between this mother and baby going. This was a clear example of the power the Chiropractic adjustment has on the nervous system and overall function of the body.

Jeanne Engert Sandheinrich, DC
1st Step Family Wellness
Whole Body Chiropractic Physician
www.1stepfamilywellness.com
314-805-7837 (Call or text)

All About Merri

Dr. Katherine A. Kadin

When Merri was just a few weeks old, her mom, Michelle, brought her in to see me for her first adjustment. Merri was barely functioning; they were both exhausted. We've all heard how newborns just eat and sleep—but not like this duo.

> Merri would sleep in fifteen-minute increments and then would be awake for fifteen-minute increments—all day, every day, around the clock!

This was unmanageable and destroying their ability to function! Michelle was at her wits end and desperate; literally pulling at straws for a solution.

I informed her that Merri's nervous system appeared to be irritated and misfiring. I said that while Chiropractic wasn't a cure-all, we'd proceed to examine her for the presence of nerve interferences; which I did in fact discover.

> After her first adjustment, Merri slept for forty-five minutes and the increments changed from fifteen minutes to thirty minutes at a time.

After the next visit, they became forty-five-minute intervals. After the third adjustment, Merri was sleeping in two-hour increments. In fact, when she arrived for her fifth adjustment, Merri was sleeping so deeply, that Michelle and I literally waited for her to wake up before I would proceed to check and adjust her. (I went on to adjust other patients, while little Merri slept for three hours!)

This is what can happen when the nervous system is functioning optimally.

Now, at almost three years of age, Merri still comes to get her spine and nervous system checked. She still sleeps well and is growing up to be a wonderful, joyful child!

Katherine A. Kadin, DC, DACCP
Kadin Family Chiropractic & Wellness Center, LLC
6212 Montrose Road
Rockville, MD 20852
240-430-1004
www.KadinFamilyChiro.com

How Bad Can It Get?

Dr. Julia Pinkerton

Jace was only four months old and in bad shape when his mother called us. She was at her wits' end. It had been thirty-eight days since Jace's last bowel movement, and she had exhausted all medical options. His condition was getting progressively worse, with longer and longer periods in between his bowel movements. Not only was he not pooping, but after every meal he would spit up five to ten times.

His parents took him from specialist to specialist and no one had any answers. Little Jace showed no signs of anything being wrong, not even constipation—he just wasn't pooping on his own. If they decided to pursue the medical route, their final option would be exploratory surgery.

Luckily one of their family friends was a chiropractor. He told them to take Jace to a chiropractor that specialized in pediatrics. Jace's parents were a bit skeptical, as they had never heard of chiropractors adjusting babies. But since they had been given no other option other than surgery, they took their son to the ER for an enema. It had gotten to the point where his body just couldn't take it any longer.

When they arrived at our office, Jace seemed like a perfectly happy, healthy baby. The only thing I found visually was that he had a slight swelling on the left side of his occiput, the lower portion of the back of his skull. On further examination, I found that the left side of his atlas, the top bone in his neck, was not moving properly. The skin temperature on that side of his neck was 2.2 degrees hotter alongside the atlas.

When I inquired as to how Jace was progressing with tummy time and rolling over, his mother told me he only rolled over to his left side. After I gently palpated his neck, doing a test which is known as an "atlas challenge," I put Jace on the floor to see what he would do. He turned to the right side for the very first time. His mother was so surprised! I explained to her that even a light input of movement in the right direction caused him to respond favorably. I was confident he was going to do very well under our care.

I adjusted Jace's atlas that day. After his first adjustment, he moved his bowels on his own for the first time in thirty-eight days. On his second adjustment, two weeks later, I worked on his atlas and his sacrum; his regurgitation became a thing of the past.

His parents told me that they would talk to Jace about coming in to see the chiropractor and his face would light up. He'd giggle every time. She teased that he had a crush on me, but I believe he realized the connection between his healing process and Chiropractic innately.

Jace's mom put it best when she wrote us a testimonial on what happened:

"I highly recommend taking your little one in. I mean, it was literally a miracle. My little guy probably would have had surgery to check what was wrong—when what he really needed was an adjustment!!!"

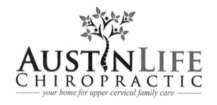

Julia Pinkerton, DC
Upper Cervical, Prenatal, and Pediatric Chiropractor
2700 W. Anderson Lane, Suite 509
Austin, TX 78757
512-452-7681
austinlifechiro.com

Honored to Care for So Many

Dr. Katie Greeley

Imagine your son, ten years old, and still wetting the bed. Imagine how emotionally difficult that must be for the parents and the child. Traditional medicine offered no real solution because the bedwetting (enuresis) was not a regular occurrence. It seemed to come and go; sometimes with too much dairy or sometimes with too much stress. Once that young boy began Chiropractic care and his nervous system started to be balanced, those bedwetting days became less and less, and eventually obsolete. The look in that child's eyes when he said, "I can now have sleepovers," brought such joy to my heart.

How about a baby with chronic recurrent ear infections? After the fifth ear infection in a six-month period, the ENT suggested ear tubes as a solution, because the antibiotics did not seem to work. Frustrated with that option, the parents looked for a less-intrusive solution. Within two months of being under Chiropractic care, the ear infections were gone; never to return that year or the next.

What if you are the parent of an eight-month-old who is not crawling yet? It only took one month of Chiropractic care for this cute, little guy to get on his fours and start moving about as if he had somewhere to go.

As a chiropractor, these are some of the many miracles I get to witness on a weekly basis. As chiropractors, we remove the interference from the nervous system and then we get to stand back and watch what nature has created. We get to see the nervous system, in all its brilliance, start to balance itself back and normal function occur.

A newborn infant comes into the office. I feel as if I have known her for nine months already, since I have been adjusting the mother since she found out her little bundle of joy was coming. Now, the little princess is here. She has been fussy for Mom and only likes to nurse on one side. After a gentle adjustment to the atlas, we see the baby stop squirming and yawn as if tension has been relieved. Later, I hear from the mother how well the baby is nursing on both sides and how well the baby is sleeping and pooping. Joy returns to baby, mother, and me.

One of the best stories I can share is about a girl lost in her own mind, diagnosed with autism. With Chiropractic adjustments, we helped her gain strength in her spine and to help her sit tall and avoid slouching; correct curves in her spine that are going the wrong way; and by doing so we were able to see her nervous system start to balance out. She started to recognize herself when she looked in the mirror, and she turned her head side to side and smiled as if she liked what she saw.

Every day I am grateful to be in a profession where I get to be a facilitator in the miracles of life. What an honor that my patients have chosen me to help guide them with their health.

Katie Greeley DC, CACCP
Certified in Family Wellness, including Prenatal and Pediatric Care
10815-3C FM 2222, Ste. 100
Austin, TX 78730
512-234-1868
www.austinwellnesschiropractic.com

SECTION THREE

Toddlers
(Bedwetting, Night Terrors)

"Chiropractors do not treat diseases, they adjust the wrong which creates disease."

B. J. Palmer, DC, The Science of Chiropractic, 1920

Miracles Help the Doctor Too!

Dr. Ali Miller

Sometimes it takes a story like this to realize that the true power of Chiropractic isn't just something you read about or hear about from someone else. Sometimes it happens to you.

The story of Baby M began with her grandmother, who had been a patient of mine for years. She understood the value of Chiropractic and referred her friends and family to me. Her most rewarding referral came in the form of a twelve-month-old beautiful girl.

Her first grandchild, Baby M was not meeting developmental milestones. Doctors told her parents that she suffered from low muscle tone and would *maybe* reach them one day. At twelve months, she could not get in or out of a sitting position on her own; she could not weight-bear on her hands and knees without crying, or her feet at all. Baby M could only finger point with her left hand, barely able to extend her right arm, and did not have pincer grasp in either hand. Her grandmother asked me if maybe Chiropractic could help.

Receiving an undeniable yes, she booked an appointment and travelled with her daughter and granddaughter to see me.

Baby M and her family had tried physiotherapy, occupational therapy, dietary changes, and multiple doctors. By the time I saw Baby M, they were at a loss about what to do next. In my office that first day, her mother regained a little hope. Although Baby M cried when I would just touch the right side of her neck, she looked at me with hope in her eyes too.

Each week, M improved dramatically. We saw her get in and out of a seated position, we saw her extend both arms and point with both hands, we saw her develop pincer grasps and we saw her CRAWL. At the end of each adjustment, as I would let Baby M know we were all done, she would cover her face and say, "Nooooo!"

At one week shy of fourteen months, Baby M put weight on her feet and finally stood with assistance. At nineteen months, Baby M walked alone! In the words of her mother:

> "After only one visit, Baby M's life was changed. Chiropractic kick-started something and allowed her body to do what it needed to do to receive the proper messages from her brain and nervous system to the development of her fine- and gross-motor skills."

Baby M is a typically developing, almost two-year-old, who runs, walks, talks and plays with her peers. With the mother's return to work and the fact they live so far away from my office, I passed on the care for Baby M to another chiropractor—but they recently came to visit me. A little diva with attitude confidently walked in but played a little shy. Although not wanting to wave to or chat with anyone in the office, when I crouched down on the floor, Baby M walked over and gave me one of the most grateful hugs I have ever received. Funny thing is, I was more grateful for having met her and being shown that I too can be a part of one of these stories.

Since a young age, Dr. Ali Miller has always had a passion for working with children. Chiropractic has given her the opportunity to enrich the families in her community with a healthy lifestyle. Her office is filled with smiles and painted handprints on the walls to bring spirit and joy to others. Dr. Ali lives in Caledon, Ontario, with her husband, Adam, and their three, well-adjusted girls, Riley, Bailey, and Zoe.

Ali Miller, DC
Family Health Chiropractic and Wellness
16 Parr Blvd. Unit 2
Bolton, Ontario
905-533-5348
www.familyhealthchiropractic.ca

You Never Know How Far-Reaching ...

Dr. Ashley Thompson

Madelyn was a beautiful five-year-old girl when her mom first brought her into my office for a consultation. She had been potty-trained for several years but had been wetting the bed nightly, a condition known as *enuresis*, and thought to be normal by many. That's certainly what Madelyn's mother thought.

When Madelyn began having difficulty making it to the bathroom in time to avoid accidents during the day, though skeptical about the value of Chiropractic care, her mother was prompted to bring Madelyn to our office.

I pride myself on always conducting a thorough consultation and examination with every patient. While taking Madelyn's history, her mother explained how Madelyn had fallen down an entire flight of stairs at seven months old. Everything appeared okay; so little attention was taken. Could that fall be the cause of Madelyn's present issues?

Upon physical examination, I noted numerous postural abnormalities and spinal subluxations. Spinal subluxations are minor displacements of the vertebrae that can lead to nervous system interference, and over time affect organ function. Once this had been explained to Madelyn's mother, I started adjusting Madelyn's spine to correct her subluxations. Her mom noticed immediate improvement. Within a short period of time, her symptoms were gone, because function had been restored and normalized.

Her mother stated: "I was very skeptical about Chiropractic and what effects it might have on Madelyn, or anyone for that matter. Today, I am a firm believer in Chiropractic care. I have even seen a great improvement in my daughter's severe sinus issues. She's had a constant runny nose for the majority of her life. Once she started getting adjusted, her nose stopped running ... Chiropractic has made it so I don't have to give Madelyn medicine for her nose."

We can all agree that an unwell child leads to difficult family dynamics, while a healthy child adds so much joy and vibrancy to a family. Madelyn and her mom consulted my office with a specific symptomatic problem, and Madelyn walked away with no symptoms, a healthier spine and nervous system, a healthy life, and so much more. We corrected the root of the problem and allowed her body to function properly.

Ashley Thompson, DC
New Beginnings Chiropractic
2290 N. Tyler, Suite 100
Wichita, KS 67205
316-721-3003
www.newbeginningswichita.com

Gavin Gordon

Dr. Chelsea Pearson

It started during the last ten days of her pregnancy. Her blood pressure increased to the point where her physician tried to induce her labor by breaking her water and giving her Pitocin. After fourteen hours of labor and two and a half hours of pushing, the baby was obviously stuck. His heart rate dropped significantly—it was obvious measures had to be taken to deliver this child.

An episiotomy and two vacuum extractions were administered to get him out quickly, resulting in a traumatic birth experience for both mother and child. The baby's head was so swollen that they kept him overnight to make sure there was no bleeding on the brain. From the onset, little Gavin struggled with nursing. He could not open his mouth fully, and Mom had to supplement his feedings. He suffered with reflux, constipation, and ear infections. A surgeon inserted tubes into his eardrums when he was twelve months old.

Gavin is now five years old and still struggles with constipation. After seeing many doctors and specialists, the only suggestion was to give him Miralax and prescription stool softeners. That was always followed with daily accidents at home and school, as well as tears and fear as a result. After continual accidents and tears, Gavin's mom brought him into the office to "try" Chiropractic.

During our first conversation, his mother revealed that he had also broken a tooth earlier this year from grinding his teeth so much at night. She said he has ground his teeth ever since his teeth came in.

My examination of Gavin revealed an elevated left shoulder and left-head tilt with a short right leg, as well as a distended tummy that pulled to his left side. He also had multiple spinal subluxations.

After the first adjustment, Gavin had a bowel movement on his own the next day. Following his fourth adjustment, he has had daily bowel movements. His mom took him off the Miralax and prescription stool softeners, and we added magnesium and probiotics to take each night before bed.

Not only is Gavin having daily bowel movements on his own, he has also stopped grinding his teeth at night. He says he now has the best sleeps. His fear of accidents has vanished and he is playing like all five-year-olds should play.

Mother and child are happy that stool softeners and medication are no longer a part of his daily routine. They are thrilled to have Chiropractic a part of his life, and Gavin looks forward to his Chiropractic visits.

Chelsea Pearson, DC, FICPA
Thrive Chiropractic
1230 N. Northwood Center Court, Suite A
Coeur d'Alene, Idaho 83814
208-665-9688
www.thrivecda.com

Nocturnal Enuresis

Dr. DoniBeth Davis

Nocturnal enuresis is something that can affect a child's life, impacting their self-esteem and social interactions. The traditional medical approach is to wait and let the child grow out of it. Most people are not aware that Chiropractic care can be helpful for children who suffer from this condition. Chiropractic adjustments allow for the nerves supplying the bladder to function properly and therefore the incidences of wetting the bed at night decrease or resolve completely.

I have had the pleasure of helping many children with this issue; I think of one boy in particular who benefited greatly from Chiropractic care.

I started seeing Carl when he was five. Around three years of age, he was able to potty train easily; however he continued to suffer from nocturnal enuresis. His mother also reported he suffered from chronic congestion and was worse with seasonal changes.

Upon examination, I was able to locate subluxations at the sacrum, T3, and upper cervical area. We began treatment. After three visits, there was a significant decrease in the number of nights he would wake up wet. He could have four nights in a row of staying dry. By the fifth treatment, Carl was able to have a two-week stretch without any incidences of nocturnal enuresis. He continued to improve and no longer has accidents at night.

I continued to see Carl on a wellness frequency. The chronic congestion continued to persist and became significantly worse in the spring. We discussed supplementation and ways to naturally support his immune system. He started to take a supplement in late summer and was able to go through the entire fall season without any aggravation of his allergy symptoms.

It has been such a joy to watch his health improve with Chiropractic care. I love being able to work with families and see the changes that happen. The success that occurs with simple, expertly delivered, noninvasive Chiropractic adjustments is always amazing. I also think about the emotional impact this has had on Carl's life, as he no longer has to deal with the insecurities caused by nocturnal enuresis.

Chiropractic works!

DoniBeth Davis, DC
Sozo Chiropractic
3720 72nd Avenue
Kenosha, WI 53144
262-764-9301

How Damaging is Bedwetting?

Dr. Kimberly Harper

This story begins in my first year of practice. At that point, I hadn't had much experience with pediatric patients.

I came into the exam room to find a grandmother sitting with her seven-year-old granddaughter Sophie, who didn't look up when I greeted her. I assumed Sophie was shy; so I did my best to make her comfortable.

The grandmother told me that Sophie had started wetting the bed a few weeks ago and her parents were exasperated trying to figure out why. She was seen by a medical doctor, a psychologist, given medicine, and made to sleep on a pad that went off like an alarm if she wet, but nothing seemed to be helping.

Sophie sat and just stared at the floor, looking embarrassed and ashamed as her grandmother told me what she had been through. Grandma mentioned Chiropractic to Sophie's parents when the problem first began, because as a child she had been under Chiropractic care for various health issues and always had positive results. The parents were skeptical of what a chiropractor could do for their daughter, but after nothing else they tried seemed to work, they finally agreed to let the grandmother bring Sophie to have her spine and nervous system checked by a chiropractor.

The history revealed that Sophie had a bad crash on her bicycle a few weeks earlier; and now that she thought about it, it was following this crash that the bedwetting started. A thorough spinal exam revealed that Sophie had a misalignment of her low back and tailbone, causing interference with the nerves controlling bladder function.

We started working with Sophie, adjusting her spine to

correct the misalignment. Sophie was always very shy and quiet during her visits. She rarely spoke to me and never looked me in the eye.

Then, one day when she was scheduled to come in, a little girl came skipping down the hall of my office with the biggest smile I had ever seen. I almost didn't recognize her; it was Sophie! She came right up to me and hugged my legs so tight I nearly fell over. She started telling me how she hadn't had any accidents since she saw me last and she was all better.

This shy, embarrassed little girl was now back to her bubbly, excited seven-year-old self. Her grandmother was also excited and continued to go on about how she knew Chiropractic could help Sophie. After just a few adjustments, what some might call a "Chiropractic miracle" occurred.

We continued to check her spine regularly and she never wet the bed again. Sophie continued to be a bright, bubbly child.

I find it so amazing how much a normal-functioning body can impact not only a person's health but also their state of mind. I am so grateful to be a chiropractor.

Kimberly Harper, DC
Family Care Chiropractic
Fishers, IN 46038
www.familycarechiro.net

The Walking Boy

Dr. Linnea Person

It was a cold, snowy Saturday morning in January; as usual, my initial thoughts when awakening were: "Ahh … Saturday morning. I don't really want to go into work on Saturdays, but when I get there, I have so much fun taking care of the people who can't come during the week." So, I jumped out of bed and got ready to serve another Saturday crowd.

About an hour after arriving at the office, a very nice mom and dad walked in carrying twenty-two-month-old Caleb. They explained that he was breech at birth, had low amniotic fluid, and ended up being a Cesarean section delivery.

By his tenth month, his mother expressed her concerns about his delayed motor skills to his pediatrician. Caleb was tested for "everything under the sun" by many specialists, with no clear answer. He was also examined at Shriners' Hospital in Chicago, and was diagnosed with a mild case of Cerebral Palsy. After a Botox injection on his spastic leg muscles, they provided braces for little Caleb to wear.

Later, his parents took him to a local chiropractor in Chicago and saw some improvement. Because one of my receptionists was a good friend of the mother, they drove the two hours to my small farming town to see if I had any suggestions for Caleb.

Caleb was held by his dad and "walked" on his toes into my exam area. The first thing I noticed was that Caleb's cranial bones (skull bones) appeared fixated, especially on the left side of his head. He also had lower-cervical spine (neck area) and lower-lumbar (low-back area) issues that required adjusting.

My initial concern was the position of his cranial bones. Mom said he'd not had them worked on before. I adjusted

Caleb based on my exam findings and suggested he return in one week.

At his second appointment, Mom said Caleb's daycare workers were amazed how improved he was; he was starting to take a few steps before he fell down. By mid-February, after just a few adjustments, Caleb was "walking much better."

Caleb has become much more outgoing, and eagerly looks forward to getting adjusted. In September, he was running around the office and his mom said, smiling, "See what you have created?!" He now moves all over on his own with the occasional fall, usually when he goes through a growth spurt. Otherwise, it appears that this little boy is functioning exactly as he was designed to—perfectly.

I am so thankful for the ability to do what I enjoy and for the referral of friends to help change the lives of these little ones!

Linnea Person, DC
1301 14th Ave.
Mendota, IL 61342-1001
815-539-3011

Sleepless in Dallas

Dr. Nikki Porteus

When I met Gia, she was three years old. Other than her sparkling boots, the first thing that stood out to me was the bright-pink cast on her wrist. Upon questioning, I learned that Gia had recently broken her arm falling down the stairs in the middle of the night. For months on end, while the rest of the family was fast asleep, Gia remained wide awake. It wasn't that Gia's sleep cycle was off to where she was sleeping all day and awake all night—she literally wasn't sleeping, period.

Concerned about her daughter, Gia's mom had taken her to their general practitioner, who tried to prescribe Gia medications to make her sleep. Refusing to accept this as the best solution, Gia's mom left her general practitioner's office frustrated and hopeful that the issue would soon resolve on its own. After dealing with Gia's insomnia for a couple more weeks, her mom took her to a holistic pediatrician's office where the nurse practitioner suggested she try Chiropractic care. Without hesitation, Gia's mom called to make an appointment at our office.

Other than the recent onset of insomnia and some seasonal allergies, Gia had experienced a healthy childhood. While Gia's mom was sleep-deprived and exhausted, Gia remained a quick-witted little girl, full of personality and a wonderful vocabulary.

I performed my exam and checked Gia's full spine, where I found subluxations in her pelvis, upper-thoracic spine, and upper-cervical spine; as well as some lymph-node swelling in her neck. As soon as I laid my fingers on C1, my gut told me that this little girl needed an adjustment!

With the goal of balancing her nervous system to more of a "rest and digest" state, I performed an osseous adjustment of C1, C2, and Gia's pelvis. Having been in practice just shy of a year, I can honestly say at that point in time, this was the biggest adjustment I had ever made with a child Gia's age. I massaged Gia's swollen lymph nodes, instructed her mom to continue using the essential oils and supplements she had already been using, and recommended that she bring Gia back at the end of the week.

Four days later, Gia and her mom returned to the office, both appearing much more rested. I asked how Gia was doing and her mom informed me that Gia had slept through the night every night since her first adjustment!

Words cannot describe how amazing it felt to know that this little girl was now able to sleep and function the way she was designed to, because of an adjustment. Gia's mom told me that she doesn't know why she didn't think of bringing Gia to a chiropractor on her own, but we both chalk it up to sleep deprivation.

Gia, her mom, and her brother continue to see me regularly; and to this day, Gia continues to sleep through the night!

Nikki Porteus, DC
APEX Wellness Center
6009 Belt Line Rd., Suite 110
Dallas, TX 75254
972-392-9402
www.apexwellnesscenter.com

Zvara

Dr. Morgan Sinclair

Alick and Meranda first came to our office because of a friend's recommendation, who was also a patient. Little did they know their lives would soon change. They, like most people, associated Chiropractic to help symptoms like headaches and lower-back pain; however, they came to us for something entirely different.

Alick and Meranda arrived at their first appointment with their three-year-old daughter, Zvara, in tow. Zvara is afflicted with Cockayne syndrome—a rare genetic disorder that prevents her from building muscle mass due to growth failure, has left her with a severely impaired nervous system, and forces her to combat premature aging. Cockayne syndrome is so rare that mainstream medical treatment options and answers are hard to come by.

Upon first meeting Zvara, she weighed in at merely eight pounds. Her parents couldn't remember one time their baby girl was able to sleep through the entire night, and her constant discomfort caused her to fall into frequent crying spells.

As she aged without growing, their emergency hospital visits increased to a minimum of once a week. Zvara received the bulk of her sustenance through a feeding tube due to her significant digestive issues. In addition to being diagnosed with scoliosis, her neck was always positioned downward, not unlike a rag doll, with no muscle mass or strength to lift her head.

After hearing "the Chiropractic story," her parents came in search of a "miracle"; although they hesitated to label it as such. They felt that as long as they went in unattached to outcomes and not expecting significant change, they couldn't lose.

Today they maintain that the power of a Chiropractic adjustment keeps them in constant amazement.

After only three months of regular Chiropractic care with Dr. Morgan, Alick and Meranda report that Zvara is now taking at least 20 percent of her food in solid form and she has doubled her daily water intake. She is finally able to lift her head up and look forward. In fact, she rarely looks down now that she can look up!

Zvara's body doesn't tremble or shake anymore and she is learning to stand and has frequent intervals when she can briefly do so on her own. Today she is a smiling, happy child who sleeps well through the night without the same level of discomfort that plagued her before this Chiropractic journey.

In the three months since starting regular Chiropractic adjustments, the family has not made any emergency visits to the hospital. And at a routine follow-up visit with her specialists, the doctors were pleased to announce that Zvara now requires far fewer appointments based on her continued progress. Seeing the remarkable transformation her daughter has undergone, Zvara's mother, Meranda, has also had amazing results after getting regular Chiropractic adjustments. She too sleeps better, no longer suffers from acid reflux, is free from her lifelong ankle and back pain, feels more energetic, and is actively excited about life and Chiropractic.

Her father, Alick, also describes feeling more alive with Chiropractic. His restful sleep and pain-free existence helps him walk better and stand tall with improved posture.

For a family whose life previously revolved around Zvara's illness, all have made huge strides and are finally able to enjoy their time as a family without the struggles that once impeded their joy.

Morgan Sinclair, DC
Streetsville Chiropractic
206 Queen Street South
Mississauga, ON L5M 1L3
905-826-0900
Drmorgansinclair@gmail.com
www.streetsvillechiropractic.com

Is There a Link Between Constipation and Not Crawling?

Dr. DoniBeth Davis

A mother brought her beautiful eighteen-month-old daughter to see me. The poor child had been dealing with constipation ever since she started to eat solid foods. The mother had tried doing everything possible to give her daughter relief. They had seen an osteopath; digestive specialists; and tried prune juice, flaxseed oil, and probiotics with minimal to no relief. Sometimes her episodes of constipation were so severe Ruby would wake up every hour screaming.

During the exam, I observed that Ruby was walking on her toes, which indicated an imbalance of her nervous system. While asking questions, I discovered that this child had never crawled. She skipped the crawling phase of development and went right to walking.

I educated the mother on the importance of crawling for brain and nervous system development. I gave the mom instructions to play with her daughter on the floor to encourage crawling.

After just two treatments, Ruby started having regular bowel movements without any difficulty. After the fifth visit, her mother sent me this text message:

> "I'm sorry to text you at home, but I just wanted to let you know that Ruby started crawling yesterday! And not just a little—she's crawling across rooms. I KNOW it is from her adjustments with you! She's had diapers like crazy since we saw you and I think she just has had more range of motion, comfortably. She's trying new things and exploring on her knees! I'm just so excited and thankful. So I had to tell you!"

Her mother also reported in a later conversation that when Ruby began crawling it was entirely on her own accord; she didn't need any encouragement to do it.

When her mother originally brought Ruby in, she wasn't aware of the importance of crawling. The care for her daughter went beyond just resolution of the original complaint of constipation. Not only did Ruby have an easier time going to the bathroom, which supports healthy digestive development, she also experienced great benefit for her brain development by crawling.

We are still working on the resolution of Ruby walking on her toes, but she is showing signs of improvement.

DoniBeth Davis, DC
Sozo Chiropractic
3720 72nd Avenue
Kenosha, WI 53144
262-764-9301

Molly

Dr. Renee M. Andino

My story is about a sweet girl named Molly who first came to our office as a twenty-month-old toddler. She was having multiple issues. Her mother stated that Molly had a history of colic and was currently dealing with recurrent ear infections, reflux, and sensory-processing issues. Molly was enrolled in speech therapy and occupational therapy. She was also taking daily doses of Prevacid and Zyrtec, drugs that were only offering mild relief of her symptoms. Molly's mother was also concerned about possible vestibular issues because her daughter appeared to be "clumsy for her age." She reported that Molly tripped a lot and still was not sleeping well at night. Molly's mom was understandably exhausted, and it was clear that Molly needed help.

Molly was gently adjusted in the upper part of her neck, mid-back, and sacrum. She also had a light abdominal massage and ileocecal valve release. For the first two weeks, she was adjusted twice per week; then appointments were reduced to once a week; and then once or twice per month.

Thankfully, Molly responded quickly to the Chiropractic adjustments! Her balance improved, as did her digestion. She also started sleeping better at night. This was a huge benefit, not only for Molly but for the entire family! After a couple weeks of consistent Chiropractic adjustments, we received the following email from her mother:

> "We just got back from Molly's OT appointment and our therapist was gob-smacked at her change. She couldn't stop talking about it. She is so skeptical of Chiropractic care and I told her how you guys are different, and she

is going to call you!! She wants to quiz you about the science of it all! We have such a testimony from your and Rob's care. We really believe you could change the face of Chiropractic care and wellness in Rockford! This town needs to know about your honesty and commitment to health and what you can do for them! We are so thankful and excited to see what the future holds!!"

She later posted the following testimonial on Facebook:

We finally get to cuddle our happy baby girl after 18 months of her being so uncomfortable and frustrated. My husband and I were at our wits' end, having tried everything we knew to do. Now she enjoys a car ride and has gone off her GI meds!! All of this after two weeks of Chiropractic care at Health First!

Now, more than a year later, Molly is a happy, healthy, and vibrant preschooler who is a joy to be around. She is full of energy and she jumps right up onto the adjusting table when it's her turn to get adjusted. It has been extremely rewarding to work with Molly and see her grow and continue to benefit from Chiropractic adjustments. It is kids like Molly who make my job so much fun!

Renee M. Andino, DC, DICCP
Board Certified in Chiropractic Pediatrics
HealthFirst Wellness Center
Rockford, IL
815-877-5575
healthfirstrockford.com

A Walk in the Park

Dr. Tim Wood and
Dr. Suzie Wood

Since nerve signals from the brain coordinate all of the functions in our body, if the spine is interfering with these signals or sending improper signals from its own receptors due to misalignment, called *subluxation*, it can affect how coordinated a child is, not to mention affect their development as a result!

Here are two examples of what parents reported in their children who struggled to walk properly from infancy.

Mom #1: "Within four weeks of starting Chiropractic treatments for our daughter, we noticed significant improvements in Estee's balance. I first noticed it when she climbed a full set of stairs one step at a time without using the handrail. Other indications are her improvements in hopping on one foot, spinning while dancing, and riding her bike. A person doesn't need to be experiencing pain to be a candidate for Chiropractic. Many people could be experiencing an improved quality of life by receiving Chiropractic care."

Mom #2: "There is nothing worse than watching your child struggle to do "normal" things a child does. I didn't get to watch K run or climb the playground equipment at the park at the "normal" ages. These were things out of reach for her. She has low muscle tone so it takes her longer to get enough strength to accomplish many things. K's muscles are really weak on one side. It felt like as soon as she got strong enough, she'd have a growth spurt and her muscles would have to play catch up.

"We met Tim at a park on Canada Day when K was almost

four years old. I figured we'd give Chiropractic a chance to see if something could help K—by this time, she'd had regular physiotherapy since she was less than a year old, with little results. When Dr. Tim met K, she was unable to run, walk for longer than five minutes (with special insoles), or climb the stairs using both feet without using a handrail.

"We began the heavy-duty process of driving in from Vernon three times a week. Within the first two months, K was able to go up and down the stairs by herself, without using a handrail. That made me nervous, but she was getting stronger.

"Now, at the end of the fourth month, she is running. She asks me if she can run everywhere. I never thought I'd have so much joy at watching a child run. I have noticed her energy increase. For the first time, I had to ask K to settle down! She is involved in everything. Before she would be quietly sitting on the couch reading, now she has a book under her arm as she runs to catch up to her siblings.

"She is more confident and sure of herself. She used to say, 'I'm too little'; now she says, 'Let me do it!'

"On Halloween, we watched K run, leading the gang from house to house. She was out for an hour. Last year, we had to push her in a stroller and often carried her up the steps because she couldn't do it. She was so excited to be involved and was quite animated in telling us about everything when she got back to Nana's.

"I am truly grateful for the practice that Dr. Tim has. Thank you for taking time out of your Canada Day."

One of the most rewarding experiences I have had in practice was seeing this girl, about eight years after she was under care. I was at a summer Bible camp with my family and all week I got to watch K playing sports, being full of life and vitality, with a smile on her face. Her parents were quick to point out how different her life would be if she had never been under Chiropractic care.

Tim Wood, DC and Suzie Wood, DC
Mission Family Chiropractic
#10 – 3818 Gordon Dr.
Kelowna, BC V1W 4V1
250-712-0900
www.missionchiropractic.ca
info@missionchiropractic.ca

Regular Sleep is Important

Dr. DoniBeth Davis

The problem with a baby that does not sleep well, is that it affects the entire family. The stress of day-to-day activities for parents is higher when they are not getting adequate sleep, which is why I especially love helping babies with sleep issues: it provides a better quality of life for the whole family.

One baby that particularly stands out from my years of practice was a fourteen-month-old boy, who had been waking frequently in the night since he was four months old. Prior to that, he had slept through the night. In the last few months, he had started to wake with night terrors. His mother was distraught and could not understand what was going on with her baby. It was difficult to calm him down once he awoke in a terror.

From what his mother could recall, nothing significant had happened at four months of age. They had consulted the pediatrician many times, with no relief.

Upon examination, I found a subluxation at C1 and his sacrum, the areas correlating with the parasympathetic nervous system which controls rest and digestion. Posture evaluation showed a right-head tilt with right-head rotation and left leg length deficiency. Adjustments were done at the areas of subluxations.

Immediately, the night terrors stopped; and if he woke up, it was much easier to get him back to sleep. With continued treatment, the frequency of his awakened nights decreased. After two months of Chiropractic care, he had made significant improvement but was not holding his adjustments as well as I would have liked. Also, he was not walking on his own—and was now sixteen months old.

I recommended he receive an evaluation from a physical therapist. The evaluation showed a weakness of the muscles on his left side. They started treatment with the physical therapist, doing the recommended exercises at home. Within a couple weeks of the PT care, he began to walk. He also started to hold his adjustments better.

In this situation, I loved how Chiropractic care and PT complemented each other so well. This collaboration allowed this sweet little boy to achieve developmental milestones and an improved quality of life. After he slept through the night for the first time, I remember his mom saying to me, "I just want to give you a hug and thank you so much for helping him and letting me get some sleep."

Sleep is such an important aspect of achieving a healthy lifestyle; rest helps make the stress of life more manageable. I love helping babies sleep through the night—so the entire family can be healthier.

DoniBeth Davis, DC
Sozo Chiropractic
3720 72nd Avenue
Kenosha, WI 53144
262-764-9301

I Love Chiropractic!

Dr. Heather L. Giesen

I had been working with a patient, who is also a mother, for about six months. After one of her appointments, she asked, "Can Chiropractic help my daughter sleep better?"

I gave her the answer I give to anyone who asks if Chiropractic can help with something in particular: "I don't know." The Chiropractic story is fairly simple. Our nervous system controls and coordinates all the cells, muscles, tissues, and organs in our body; thus coordinating every function it needs to perform. I explained, "If a bone in your daughter's spine is out of alignment, or subluxated, and hindering how her nervous system functions, it could also hinder your daughter's ability to completely relax and stay asleep at night."

She described to me that her one-and-a-half-year-old, Brynn, was a poor sleeper and had never slept through the night. Every night she wakes up; usually between the hours of 1:00 and 4:00 a.m.

It is tough waking up with a baby every night and still find the energy to function during the day. Now, imagine you also have a three-year-old at home too. The parents were exhausted!! When you lack sleep, it's easy to get frustrated; not only at your children, but also at each other and all the people you need to communicate with during the day.

After our conversation, she decided it couldn't hurt to make an appointment to have Brynn checked for a subluxation. At her first appointment, we did a consultation and an exam consisting of posture analysis and a thermography scan. After a thorough analysis, it was obvious a subluxation was present in Brynn's sacrum and at the second cervical vertebra, called C2. I had to work with Brynn, like many busy toddlers who haven't been adjusted before, to get her to sit still long enough to adjust her. Her mother and I gently worked together, and I was able to adjust her S2 while she was lying on her tummy and her C2 was adjusted while she was sitting on her mom's lap.

After a couple adjustments, I recognized that something was changing. When they came for their appointment, Brynn would give me signs that she was ready for her turn. Her mother would hold her while I ran my nervoscope, and she sat very still to let it happen.

After a handful of adjustments, I heard the words I was waiting to hear: "She has been sleeping through the night." After a year and a half of interrupted sleep, imagine how much better life is for Brynn and the rest of the family!

Heather L. Giesen, DC, CACCP
Giesen Family Chiropractic
815 1st Street SE, New Prague, MN 56071
952-758-8760
"For Pediatric Development to Adult Health"
www.giesenfamilychiropractic.com

SECTION FOUR

Children and Teens
(Migraines, Falls, Sports Injuries)

"At the heart of Chiropractic is the spinal adjustment. The chiropractor, in attempting to restore and maintain optimum health, locates and corrects spinal subluxations to enhance nervous-system function. This corrective process is called a *spinal adjustment.*"

GILLES A. LAMARCHE, DC

Aiden

Dr. Dennis Mizel

I have had the honor of serving people in my home city of St. Catharines, Ontario, Canada, for thirty-eight years. My career has been filled with a cascade of love and joy. More than anything else, taking care of young children brings immense satisfaction.

Chiropractic is one of the best-kept secrets in the world! It has become clear to me that Chiropractic is an essential health care profession. Chiropractic care can be best understood by gaining clarity on three universal laws:

1. The body is a self-healing organism. When you cut your finger, your body goes through a cascade of processes to heal itself.

2. The nervous system (brain, spinal cord, and nerves) is our master control system that controls, coordinates, and regulates every system, every organ, and every cell in our bodies.

3. Vertebral subluxation interferes with our master control system.

It must be understood that vertebral subluxation chokes off life, and the longer there is interference present, the weaker the cells, organs, and systems of the body become. Chiropractors are the only health-care practitioners trained to locate and correct vertebral subluxation.

Aiden was four years and four months old when he first attended my office. He was in Junior Kindergarten and was a very active boy. He was a middle child, having an eight-year-old brother and seven-month-old sister.

Aiden complained of calf cramps, with pain in both left and right leg every night that extended from his knees to his ankles. His condition had persisted for eight months. His mother advised that the pain was so intense he cried nightly. She would massage his calves and give him Tylenol. This home remedy did not alter the nightly event of calf pain and crying, but it did appear to afford Aiden some relief.

A Chiropractic assessment identified limited motion on standing, and leaning to the left compared to leaning to the right. Vertebral subluxation was identified at his mid back and upper aspect of his lower back. A treatment plan was developed. Aiden was instructed to have his spine checked and corrected, if needed, twice per week for six weeks and then once per week for twelve weeks.

Aiden responded well to Chiropractic treatment. After one week, his mother reported he had three nights without any cramps. By the third week, he no longer had cramps. He continued per our recommended schedule for the full eighteen weeks and had leg cramps only once more during that period. Although I recommended Aiden continue on a maintenance schedule of once per month, his mother preferred she bring him in as needed.

I next saw Aiden eighteen months later. His mother advised he had a new three-week bout of wetting the bed and wondered if Chiropractic could help. She also advised that the children can be rough with one another and that Aiden had complained of some low-back pain a month earlier for a week's duration that she managed with home massage.

When his lower-back pain improved, the bedwetting began. Bedwetting was a challenge for six-year-old Aiden. Although he didn't say a word, it was clear he was concerned. There was embarrassment and concerns about sleepovers. He refused to go to a friend's house for a sleepover, which had never been a concern in the past.

Our assessment revealed vertebral subluxation at various levels. Our treatment plan was to see Aiden twice per week for six weeks and then once a week for twelve weeks; and then re-evaluate. After one visit, he had a dry night. He was dry from that day forward and he continues to be seen monthly on a preventative maintenance schedule of care to keep his nervous system functioning as well as it can. Aiden and his mother both understand that the nervous system controls, coordinates, and regulates every system, organ, and cell in our bodies. A nervous system that functions well affords us the best health possible.

I am so lucky that I was chosen to be a chiropractor. I know it sounds like a cliché, but when asked what the greatest career in the world is, I know with certainty that I would choose every day to be a chiropractor!

Dennis Mizel, DC
St. Catharines Chiropractic & Health Centre
320 Vine Street
St. Catharines, ON L2M 4T3
905-934-7776
www.stcatharineschiropractic.com

The Marvel Never Ceases

Dr. Colin Henderson

The local office of a large national company invited me to be a part of their annual health fair. Each employee was given a "passport" and had the opportunity to speak with a massage therapist, a nutritionist, me, and other health care providers. Each stamp on their passport got them an entry into a draw for some awesome prizes. I spoke to over sixty people during the two-hour event.

KL, despite knowing since childhood that she had a significant scoliosis, had never been to a chiropractor. She had never even spoken with one. I had no idea of any of this as I shared the principle of Chiropractic with her and a small group of her coworkers. She immediately made an appointment for herself and her son.

"I'd love it if you could help me, but I'm really worried about my son," she said.

> "His posture is terrible and he gets headaches all the time. He also has anxiety, panic attacks, and periods of severe depression. He's on several medications, including some really powerful antidepressants, and he's been struggling like this for several years. I'm just worried sometimes he might hurt himself."

When KL came for her initial visit, her son, M, was not with her. He had been admitted to an in-patient care facility because his depression had gotten dangerously severe. Amazingly, M made this admission possible himself. He knew he needed help. He had been missing a lot of school simply because he couldn't get out of bed. He was only sixteen.

Through tears, KL explained what had happened leading

up to his admission. His entire life hung in the balance of life or death. He spent over a month in that facility; and yes, it saved his life, but for what?

When M finally came in to see me, his posture was so bad that his height measured at 6'1" even though his mother wrote 6'4" on the intake form. He barely made eye contact and his answers were short and lifeless. He didn't smile or laugh; he shifted side to side in his seat. Just being in our office made him anxious and uncomfortable.

During the exam, I reflected on what was possible for this young man. I gave them hope. They scheduled a review visit for the following day. I broke down and cried when they left. It was one of the most difficult exams I've ever completed. I prayed that I would get a chance to lay my hands on this young man.

M started getting adjusted four times a week, and it took two weeks before he even made eye contact with me. The first three months were up and down for M. Some days he'd come in and smile at my dumb jokes; and other days, he'd just go through the motions of getting adjusted. I could tell he was healing but it was a tough go for him.

After six months of care, when we did his progress exam, M checked off so many improvements on the review form I just about screamed: fewer headaches; less neck pain; better immune system; sleeping better; more alert; and, best of all, less depression and anxiety, and more positive attitude and no panic attacks.

Within six months, M was a different person. He smiled and had conversations with me. He had goals for school and was again active with his family on the weekends.

M has been under our care for two years, and now has excellent posture. He laughs a lot and is doing great in school. He has decreased the medications he's on and we think he'll be drug-free someday. He's had a few anxiety and panic attacks in the past eighteen months and only one significant period of depression in the last year. He is much better able to recognize what's happening inside before it really takes off.

M said, "I feel much more like me now. All the heaviness is gone."

In a private conversation with his Mom, she told me, "I feel like my little boy is back."

We both cried and marveled at the healing that has happened for him. Then, we both laughed at the thought of her now 6'7" boy being described as "little."

Colin Henderson, DC
Marda Loop Family Chiropractic
2110A – 33 Avenue SW
Calgary, AB T2T 1Z7
403-217-3002
www.livelifewell.ca

The Happy Accident

Dr. Deborah A. Fudge

Randy was involved in a serious car accident and, as a result, developed sharp lower-back and leg pain. He consulted with me for Chiropractic care and started seeing improvement in his health after a month of treatment.

One day, when Randy came into the office, he was fit to be tied. Aisling, his twelve-year-old daughter, had to be picked up from school due to an excruciating migraine. She had been getting debilitating headaches and migraines for over five years. Randy and Aisling's mom had taken her to her pediatrician. She had seen the top neurologist in Boston, and had every test imaginable performed, including a CT scan, an MRI, and blood tests. Aisling was prescribed medication, which helped marginally, but caused severe weight gain. Needless to say, Randy was frustrated that his only child continued to suffer.

I asked him if any of the specialists had recommended a chiropractor, which they had not. I explained to Randy that sometimes headaches can be caused from problems in the neck; I encouraged him to bring Aisling in for a consult.

"Not seeing her in pain anymore—that's all I care about. I can see in her eyes when she's hurting, and it kills me," he said.

When Randy brought Aisling in for her first appointment, I could tell she was nervous. I explained to them that I would be checking her spine for subluxations, vertebrae that could be out of alignment disrupting the communication between her brain and body and body to brain. My goal was to remove any interference with that communication.

After our consult, I examined her spine and took X-rays of her neck. As I was palpating the area right below her skull, she winced and said, "This is where my headaches start." She paused and said, "I just want my life back and to have a day without a headache."

I showed Randy and Aisling what a normal cervical X-ray should look like and then I showed them her X-rays. It was obvious to twelve-year-old Aisling that something wasn't right in her neck. Her atlas, the top vertebra in the spine, was wedged up below her skull. I explained that this was the main cause of her headaches.

Randy had a look that any parent would recognize: *hope*. He was relieved that his daughter would no longer have to live in pain every day.

After only three weeks of Chiropractic care, Aisling has had only two headaches, compared to once daily migraines. She is now able to dance and read easily, her focus has improved at school, and she no longer needs pain medication. We have addressed some lifestyle changes, which have been helpful when she feels stressed.

"It's unbelievable how a car accident turned into getting rid of my daughter's headaches!" said Randy during a recent appointment.

Stories like Aisling's continue to inspire me as a chiropractor. It is an honor and a blast going to work every day. I feel blessed to have the privilege of helping people get their lives back in a drug-free and natural way.

Dr. Deborah Fudge is a family based chiropractor serving Methuen, MA and the Merrimack Valley area for thirty years. She is a graduate of the Palmer College of Chiropractic in Davenport, Iowa. Dr. Fudge's personal life statement is to bring love and peace everywhere she goes and to make a difference to one new person every day.

Deborah A. Fudge, DC
76 Woodland St.
Methuen, MA 01844
978-686-7791
www.drdebfudge.com
facebook.com/drdebfudge

Jeremy's Plight

Dr. Michael Gaitonde

When I first met Jeremy, he was seven years old and had been struggling with a tremor for nearly five years. His mom described it like trying to change the radio when you hit a speed bump. The tremor made otherwise simple tasks, like brushing his teeth and eating, acts of endless frustration. While the rest of Jeremy's classmates were beginning to perfect their writing skills, his handwriting remained nearly illegible. When Jeremy and his younger siblings brought coloring to the office, Jeremy's work lacked the precision that was in his siblings' drawings. Having dealt with this nearly his whole life, Jeremy saw these things as "normal," but exasperating nonetheless.

Pursuing every avenue to find a solution to his mysterious ailment, Jeremy's parents sought the expertise of multiple doctors, neurologists, and professionals at Johns Hopkins University. After tests, blood work, and MRIs, the doctors could only recommend medication to potentially minimize the issue. After doing some online research, his parents decided to try Chiropractic as a last resort—unfortunately the reason why many people seek out chiropractors.

When I first met the family, they were understandably nervous and wary of discovering yet another dead-end. After assessing Jeremy, I found he had hypertonicity in his arms that was affecting his fine-motor skills. I suspected that Jeremy's issues were linked to birth trauma from an emergency C-section. His mother explained that the umbilical cord was wrapped around his tiny, fragile neck three times.

"As the twig is bent, so grows the tree," aptly describes Jeremy's situation. His suppressed nervous system affected his fine-motor skills and after seven years of this underlying issue going unaddressed, the impact appeared permanent.

Jeremy was standoffish at first, but allowed me to work on his spine. He proved to be curious about the science behind his treatment, always asking questions about how the body worked. Eventually, the conversation turned from science to Legos and iPad games. As I got to know Jeremy, I got to know the entire family, and soon everybody was getting adjusted.

I retested Jeremy's handwriting after three months of treatment and the results showed remarkable improvement. Not only had the tremor dramatically decreased, but Jeremy now exuded a calm confidence. His renewed control over his body opened him up to a world of possibilities. Everyday tasks were no longer insurmountable obstacles to overcome. Jeremy could eat, brush his teeth, and write much more easily. He also enjoyed expressing creativity, bringing in drawings and comics to show off his new skills.

Witnessing Jeremy's transformation has left a positive mark on my heart and my career. After three years of care, I can confidently say that Jeremy has seen measurable improvement. The tremor has for the most part disappeared, and if you look at his handwriting today you could never tell he had a problem. Today, Jeremy has renewed confidence and control over his abilities, and his struggles have taught him determination and perseverance.

Throughout Jeremy's time as my patient, I performed spinal adjustments with no additive therapy. His progress exemplifies the undeniable power of correcting spinal subluxations, allowing the nervous system to work as it was meant to perform.

Michael Gaitonde, DC
Lighthouse Chiropractic
7310 Heritage Village Plaza
Gainesville, VA 20155
www.lighthousechiro.com

St. Lucia

Dr. Sharon Goodyear

We were on a family vacation in St. Lucia. My two boys and I were playing at the resort's castle. It was a small building with two stories joined by a spiral cement staircase. Ocean breezes wafted through the window openings. It was a delightful time.

I was one step behind my two-and-a-half-year old, Liam, who was slowly descending the stairs. In front of Liam, a young boy of approximately five years was running full tilt down the steps, gaining space with each moment. Most of my attention was on Liam's efforts when the other boy fell. He went down hard on his butt on the edge of the bottom step. His mother came around the corner in time to observe the impact but too late to intervene.

The child looked at his mom and then went slack. He did not make a sound. She scooped him up and carried him to a nearby bench.

Liam and I approached the bench as Mom was starting to freak out. The boy had lost consciousness. I had witnessed the way the boy had landed and knew that he had most likely injured his spine. His head had not hit the steps.

I told the mom I was a chiropractor and asked if I could check her son's spine. I was confident that a Chiropractic adjustment could help, and she responded to that confidence. (Later I found out she had absolutely no idea what a chiropractor was or what we did.) As indicated by a quick check, I adjusted his pelvis and upper neck. Two tiny, gentle adjustments.

She looked at me with wide eyes; her hands came up in front of her with palms open, and she said, "That's it?" with some agitation in her voice.

155

"Yup, that's it." I began to doubt myself and started to try and think of what else I could do. All of this happened in slow-moving seconds, enough time for a small group of children and parents to wander over.

At that moment, her son started to open his eyes. His lids raised and only the whites of his eyes were visible at first. Then, he sat up, looked at his mom, and asked, "What happened?" He was obviously a bit confused.

Once he noticed he was the center of attention, he started to cry and buried his face in his mom's chest. By now, both she and I were also crying from relief.

Before we parted, I made arrangements to check her son's spine again. Over the next few days, we chatted and Mom told me that when her son was lying there unconscious, she was trying to figure out how she could get him home to England to get medical attention. Her imagination had projected into a future with possible permanent repercussions from that fall.

As a thank-you, she gave me a small painted pot made from a local island gourd. It is blue with lovely, brilliant-colored flowers on it. That pot still sits on my dresser to remind me to never doubt the healing power of a Chiropractic adjustment.

Sharon Goodyear, DC
Bruce Street Family Chiropractic
81 Bruce St., Kitchener ON N2B 1Y7
519-743-6339
drsharon@brucestreetfamilychiropractic.com

Two Brothers

Dr. Sue Mullen

In June 2015, Tabatha, a mother of five children, skeptically started Chiropractic care with me. After she felt amazing results with her own health, she asked if I would examine two of her sons. Her intuition and my recommendations paid off.

At four years old, Rome had fallen and fractured his skull. An MRI revealed a Chiari Malformation of his cranium. It was subsequently surgically repaired using parts of his Atlas and Axis. After his recovery from surgery, his parents noticed his temperament had changed. He was no longer the happy-go-lucky and fun-seeking child he once was. He would have unwarranted and random temper outbursts and severe mood swings. His digestion became abnormal and he was cranky most of the time. Needless to say, his parents were perplexed and concerned. Medical doctors offered drugs, but they said no.

Rome started Chiropractic care two years after his surgery. He again became a fun-loving and energetic child with no digestive issues and no senseless outbursts.

His twelve-year-old brother, Tristin, had had a difficult birth. Before Chiropractic care, he was sensitive and irritated whenever anyone touched his neck or when anything was around his neck. He would struggle to free even the mildest of restraints. He couldn't run very fast or for very long. His X-rays revealed agenesis of the posterior arch of Atlas. (My question to other chiropractors is: why would you not X-ray a child?)

With Chiropractic care, Tristin feels more like a normal child, running with his classmates and friends.

He stated, "I am now more available and willing to do things that I am not normally good at. I feel different emotionally and physically. I love coming to see Dr. Sue."

This family went from being total Chiropractic skeptics to enthusiastic wellness converts.

Sue Mullen, DC
The Good Life Chiropractic
2620 Telegraph Avenue
Berkeley, CA 94704
510-356-4048
www.thegoodlifechiropractic.com

From Severe Pain to Full Recovery

Dr. Todd Watson

My name is Alyssa Leblanc. I live in Huntsville, a small town in Northern Ontario, Canada. When I was eleven years old, I was diagnosed with suspected Fibromyalgia. I was having severe low-back pain that would sometimes shoot up to my middle back.

My mother took me to see our medical doctor in Huntsville, who then referred me to a pediatrician in Orillia, but no one could tell us what was wrong with me.

I could not do anything other kids could do. I could not ride on the school bus and my parents had to drive me to school every day. I could not play with my friends or do phys-ed. I had to bring a pillow to school to sit on and I felt embarrassed. We tried physiotherapy, with no help. I went to the chiropractor, which helped for a little while, but then the pain came back. We tried massage, swimming, and medications called naproxen and Robaxacet. Nothing seemed to help.

One day, the pain was getting so bad my parents drove us three hours to Toronto and took me to the Emergency Room at Sick Kids Hospital. The doctor in Emergency put me on Toradol and referred me to a pediatric neurologist at Sick Kids. I was then referred to a genetic specialist. When they said they could find nothing wrong with me, they referred me to a back specialist at Mt. Sinai Hospital. He sent me to the Bloorview MacMillan Rehab Centre, where I stayed for five weeks doing rehabilitation for my back.

The pain was being managed by using Toradol, but when I got back from rehab, it started up again, even with the medication. We didn't know what to do next. We felt we had tried everything. It didn't seem normal for a kid my age to be taking pain medications every day.

One of my parent's friends recommended we see Dr. Todd Watson in Huntsville. We were doubtful, as we had tried Chiropractic and it helped for only a little while.

In Dr. Watson's office, everyone was helpful and encouraging. Dr. Jocelyn examined me and she was very gentle and kind, which was good because it was so painful to do the tests. Dr. Watson insisted on taking his own X-rays as he said that the ones I had taken previously were taken lying down and he wanted standing X-rays.

We returned two days later to see the results of my examination. Dr. Watson showed my mom and me that I had a short leg on one side, which was causing my spine to curve out of normal alignment. He told me I needed to put a heel lift in my shoe and take a series of Chiropractic adjustments.

The first few days of treatment, I was very sore, but by the end of seven days I WAS PAIN FREE! I am now doing all the normal things a kid can do—and do not take any medications.

My mother told Dr. Watson that if Chiropractic worked for me, she would come in and kiss his feet. He assured her that was not necessary.

Todd Watson, DC
Advanced Chiropractic Clinic
www.forwardheadposture.ca

Parenting with Leadership

Dr. John Filo

As a parent of three girls, I want the best for my children. Every parent wants the best for their child; they want their child to be happy and healthy. When health and happiness are absent, we–as parents–are called to action. Immediately.

When parents notice something is wrong, we take action without hesitation, whether it's a challenge at school or with homework, a social conflict with friends, or fighting a cold and flu. Whatever the challenge, a parent steps up. It's our duty, our obligation. "Nothing will get in the way of providing care and support for MY child!" you say.

But what if urgency is not present? What if an alarm doesn't sound off? What if we think everything is fine and little Johnny is doing okay in school? He sleeps well. He's eating okay; nothing out of the ordinary. What is our duty as a parent then?

It's a question we rarely ask ourselves. We fail to ask this question because we fail to recognize the fact that leaders are not born, leaders are developed.

What I'm talking about is the role of a parent in the development, nurturing, and honing of their child's God-given potential. It requires an understanding that leadership is not something you're born with; the same way an Olympic Gold Medalist is not born a champion. It is developed.

The development of a leader starts from within.

As parents, we have access to the seed of that potential. I believe parents have an obligation and duty to ensure that seed is nurtured. I believe our job is to identify the nature of that seed, the unique strength of that seed, and to guide and support it through its development. That's the attention a parent who understands leadership brings into the space of parenting.

And it starts with the most primary of all functions, the brain and nervous system. The interface between the body and the environment is the nervous system. It determines one's state of mind; how one perceives reality. It determines one's functional capacity; how one's movement, balance, strength, and agility are harnessed. It determines one's rate of regeneration and how one heals and replenishes vital life force.

The nervous system is the impetus of development. To be a leader is to be fully engaged, to be present, and to be in a state of readiness.

This is the essence of a Chiropractic adjustment, not for pain relief, not even for injury prevention. It is the understanding that the brain and nervous system are the keys to development and peak performance. They are the keys to developing leadership in our children.

When Chiropractic is sought for this reason and combined with a healthy and wholesome dietary regimen, physical activity, and creative expression, then parenting is taken to another level.

Parents who understand this concept are in a different realm. They are no longer reacting to struggle and challenge. They are proactively taking ownership to ensure the child has every opportunity to express his/her pure potential.

This is parenting with leadership.

John Filo, DC
Yonge Finch Chiropractic & Health Centre
5650 Yonge Street, Suite 1A
Toronto, ON M2M 4G3
www.yongefinchhealth.com
drjfilo@gmail.com

Londyn

Dr. Sharon Goodyear

I first met Londyn when she was a few months old. Jo was her foster mom at the time and she brought Londyn in with her whenever she was having her regular spinal check and adjustment. By the time Londyn was two, Jo had completed the adoption process and we started doing regular spinal checks and adjustments on Londyn too.

On a Wednesday in August 2015, our office received a frantic call from Jo. Londyn had been injured at the local water park and they were on their way over from the hospital.

The usually high-energy three-year-old was carried in and sat on my table. There was none of her usual exuberance; no "Hi Dr. Sharon"; no small arms stretched up for her welcome hug.

She had been accidentally knocked over by an older boy and had her full face planted on the cement deck. Neither Jo nor her Aunty Joy had seen Londyn's hands come up to break the fall. Her sullen look was marked by a swollen and cut upper lip and nose, her eyes were bloodshot, and bruising was starting to come out under her eyes. It was determined at the hospital that there was no bony fractures but everyone expected huge raccoon eyes by morning.

When I checked Londyn's spine it indicated to adjust the very top of and midway down her neck (C1 and C5). I adjusted her while she sat on her mother's lap, legs wrapped around her waist and her head draped over Jo's shoulder.

They left with instructions to come back Thursday and Friday morning.

Londyn bounced in Thursday. All smiles and hugging arms. Jo's enthusiasm was contagious with everyone in the office as she shared their experience. Within thirty minutes of receiving her adjustment they (Jo and Aunt Joy) watched as the swelling and 90 percent of the redness went away from Londyn's lip and nose.

As Londyn sat on the table, there was none of the expected bruising under and around her eyes. Her lip was still tender where her teeth had punctured it, and the scratches were still visible, but the change in less than twenty-four hours was remarkable.

It was awesome that the office was full of people to hear this wonderful news! In truth, I was silenced and brought to tears observing the body's incredible ability to heal when the spine is subluxation-free. Without interference the power that made the body is free to do its job of running and regenerating that body—and it does it with perfection.

Sharon Goodyear, DC
Bruce Street Family Chiropractic
81 Bruce St., Kitchener ON N2B 1Y7
519-743-6339
drsharon@brucestreetfamilychiropractic.com

Happy Child Again

Dr. Sue Mullen

When Lydia was two years old she had two serious falls from her stroller. After the first fall, her father commented that she had changed from being a happy child to a much more discontented one. After each fall, her parents had taken her to a medical doctor and they said they did not find anything wrong with Lydia. Therefore, her parents did not think there was anything more to be done.

Lydia's mother began care in our office. After a few weeks of care, she told me of Lydia's falls and the change in her demeanor. I was anxious to examine this little girl to see if she could be helped. Her X-rays revealed her neck had been damaged from the falls.

As her father stated: "That fall really did alter her life, and in a negative way!"

Now, at seven years old, Lydia was complaining of neck pain. Her mother was more concerned about her mood swings and shifts in her energy level. Her mother said, "If it is not taken care of, it will inhibit her"; reflecting on the possibility of these bad moods and energy shifts becoming a permanent part of Lydia's personality. Her mom knew this would influence the growth and outlook of this young and precious life!

After Lydia's first Chiropractic adjustment, her mother said, "I could see right away, from the spark in her eyes, that her spirit had returned. Lydia said that the treatments were fun, and I could sense her whole organism liking this process of becoming aligned again. Her energy rapidly returned to her.

"Thanks to your Chiropractic adjustments, Dr. Sue, my daughter can truly know herself; thus learn to master herself and guide herself to her greatest potential. And my husband

and I can feel the burden of that original fall lifting. It is so wonderful to embrace our daughter as she is—more aligned with herself."

Now Lydia's father and younger brother are also under Chiropractic care.

Power on!

Sue Mullen, DC
The Good Life Chiropractic
2620 Telegraph Avenue
Berkeley, CA 94704
510-356-4048
www.thegoodlifechiropractic.com

The Plight of a Ten-Year-Old

Dr. Jeanne Engert Sandheinrich

When I met Liam, he would soon celebrate his eleventh birthday. He was a happy, smiling boy; but as soon as his mother started to talk to me about his bedwetting, his face saddened. He had been wetting the bed ever since potty training. He sadly concurred, "Ever since I can remember."

At night, he would regularly leak or completely void his bladder once or twice per week. Liam was self-conscious of this issue. I could see it on his face when I started to ask him questions about what was going on. He was active in Boy Scouts and the bedwetting deterred him from going on trips.

There was a period of time when his mother used an alarm on the bed to wake him when he started to wet. They said that it helped for about six months, but then the wetting went right back to where it was before. They were already eating a healthy gluten-free diet, limited dairy, and limited sugar. Their lifestyle seemed to be relaxed and not emotionally stressful. He and his brother were home-schooled and seemed to enjoy each other's company.

During his exam, I found that Liam's sacrum and pubic bone were not moving properly. I told him I was going to adjust him to make his body move properly, explaining that when the spine is not moving properly, or is misaligned, the nervous system cannot efficiently communicate with the rest of the body. I told him that we call a misalignment, or area of the spine that is not moving correctly, a *subluxation*. A subluxation inhibits the nervous system from correctly communicating to the rest of the body, and in his case, his subluxations appeared to be inhibiting proper function of his bladder.

Liam is very smart and got it right away. He said, "It is like a computer, controlling everything, and a pop-up window popping up and preventing you from doing your work." I was very impressed.

We started treatment right away. I adjusted his sacrum, pubic bone, and worked on the muscles and ligaments near the pubic bone. When I checked in on Liam at the next appointment, he was eager to tell me that he did wet a few times, but it was much less than usual. I adjusted him the same at this visit and told him to keep monitoring everything for me. At his third visit, prior to treatment, he told me that he did not wet the bed at all during that week. His face was lit up with joy and confidence was radiating off of him. Liam did not wet the bed any more after that treatment.

Now, almost six months later, Liam is still dry. Over the summer, he went on a weekend camping trip without having to worry about having a wet night. He was confident that he would not. Liam and his whole family are under Chiropractic care two times per month because they saw the power of the nervous system firsthand.

Jeanne Engert Sandheinrich, DC
1st Step Family Wellness
439 S. Kirkwood Rd., Suite 214
St. Louis, MO 63122
314-805-7837 (Call or text)
Pediatric & Prenatal Chiropractic Physician
www.1stepfamilywellness.com

Devastating Migraines

Dr. Jon Saunders

I will always remember the fear in her eyes when I walked into my exam room. Julie was frightened and holding back tears when she spoke. It was a busy day in the office and my assumption was she was extremely nervous about being here.

I soon learned that her terror wasn't for herself, but for her six-year-old son, who wasn't with her. She told me that her friend had pleaded with her to seek out a chiropractor for her young son who had been suffering from debilitating migraines since the age of three. Due to fear, she hadn't listened. Finally, when her fear of the unknown was trumped by her fear of a neurologist (who had told her that no one could help her son) and who had recommended daily prescription drugs with potentially serious side effects, she garnered enough courage to walk through my door.

After a nerve system exam, X-rays, and palpation of Lukas, it was clear the problem was coming from Lukas' neck. I remember telling Julie that was really quite simple, we find the cause and then we correct it. From the exam, it was very clear the nerves in the top of Lukas' neck were being irritated and choked by his upper-cervical subluxations.

She remained skeptical, which is not unusual for someone new to Chiropractic, since she had tried various other interventions to help her son—dietary changes, vitamins, and even acupuncture. I just told Julie with confidence that I had 100 percent faith that Lukas' body would heal because it is perfectly designed to do so. She trusted my conviction, and after explaining the Chiropractic principle, it made sense to her.

I truly believe if my belief in what I do wasn't resilient the morning I met Julie, Lukas would have never become a patient in my office and would have never experienced the principle of Chiropractic. Since Lukas had suffered since he was three years old, I knew it may not be an easy path to recovery, but I did know he would heal.

We started by focusing on his upper neck, with very specific, gentle adjustments. His healing happened little by little. As nerve pressure was reduced, his body healed, and he had less and less pain. He was able to participate in school activities and sports without incident.

Within nine months, Lukas' body did exactly what it was designed to do naturally: it healed. As his mom put it, "My son's migraines have virtually disappeared. His energy levels are through the roof and he is excelling academically, socially, and in a number of sports, including hockey."

Jon Saunders, DC
www.chiropracticfirst.ca

The Concerned Mom

Dr. Jonathan Diplock

On Friday, July 24, 2015, my fourteen-year-old son woke up with excruciating pain in his spine. The discomfort was to the point where he could barely breathe. As an anxious mother, my first thought was to call a chiropractor. The Chiropractic team responded to our urgency, suggesting that we bring him in immediately. The staff was very friendly and helpful as they guided us through the process of becoming a new member of their practice. The doctor began by asking questions about the area of concern but also asked questions about troubling issues of previous injuries that my son had accumulated.

During the winter of this year, my son sustained a head injury that resulted in a concussion while playing hockey. After hitting his head into the boards, he was helped off the ice and brought into the dressing room. He was evaluated by the team trainer and was told he would have to take time off for the symptoms to subside. He was not allowed to return to the game he loved.

Being a very active young man, my son did not take well to being told he had to take time off from sports. After a short while, he returned to hockey with no symptoms of headache, dizziness, or physical ailments. Everything seemed to be back to normal, at least physically. However, my mom senses knew that something had shifted and was different—his personality. I told myself that over time his jovial, excited, fun-loving self would return and that I was worrying over nothing.

Instead, my son developed into someone I did not recognize. He became short-tempered; moody; developed a poor memory; and had trouble concentrating, having the attention span of a young child. I convinced myself that this was part of him growing up and going through puberty. He just never came back to being himself. I felt odd sharing these concerns with the doctor and his team. My first thought was that they would think I was crazy or in denial, expecting the doctor to perform a Chiropractic lobotomy with a personality miracle.

As the doctor began to explain the extent of the injuries and challenges my son was having, answers started to appear about my unexplainable concerns. I have little knowledge of the nervous system and even less understanding on how it could be damaged. The doctor explained that lifestyle and injuries could create distortions of the spine and interfere with the way the nerves were supposed to work. He explained that the body is self-healing, but this was being blocked by misalignments in his spine called *subluxations*. When this was explained to me, my heart lifted. Was there still hope to regain the young man I so desperately missed?

We began having his spine corrected immediately. It was not long before the initial concerns of pain subsided. What was truly amazing, is that a few weeks later, my son started emerging from blank stares and irritation that had dominated his personality and became his normal self.

Today my family is whole again. We have joined the Chiropractic team as practice members and look forward to taking care of our health for many years. I am truly grateful for two things: that my son has been given his life back and that it was managed without the need for medication.

A truly grateful and concerned mom

Dr. Jonathan Diplock is a wellness-based chiropractor who practices out of Val Caron, Ontario, Canada. His practice is focused on the evaluation of nervous system integrity and maintaining optimal health through a neurological lens.

Jonathan Diplock, DC
Family Wellness Centre
Val Caron, Ontario P3N1N6
705-897-6711
sudburyfamilywellness@gmail.com

How Does it Feel to Have No Friends?

Dr. Kimberly Koski

Kristin is a smart, bright, energetic girl who had a serious problem that made her an outcast and the target of bullies. She first entered my office at the impressionable young age of seven. Kristin's mother explained that she heard about me from a woman at her work and I was their last resort.

Kristin's short history started with a C-section birth; colic; and severe, painful constipation. She was prescribed several types of medications. Although some helped for a short time, nothing was resolved. The problem with her bowels persisted.

As Kristin got older, she was able to tell her parents what she was experiencing. She explained that she didn't feel the need to "poo" but then it would be there in her underwear. Her pediatrician diagnosed her with a mega colon and told her parents that there was nothing they could do for Kristin other than to prescribe medication. Thankfully, her mother realized that Kristin having to take medication for the rest of her life did not seem like the best idea.

When Kristin first entered my office, she appeared to be a wonderful, happy girl and she was curious to know what I was planning to do with her. She wanted me to "fix" her.

Kristin's mother explained that she had to leave work every day at noon to help Kristin "clean up." Because Kristin could not feel the need to have a bowel movement, her underwear would be filled and consequently, Kristin would smell. The children in Kristin's class alienated Kristin and ultimately bullied her.

Kristin, although seemingly happy in my office, was a sad little girl. She was moved from one class to another to help improve the situation, to no avail.

After a full exam, it was revealed that Kristin was severely subluxated. I explained Chiropractic to her and her mother and they agreed to start care. Kristin was faithful with her adjustments and diet restrictions; and in time, we celebrated each of her accomplishments.

At first her improvement was slow, but as she continued Chiropractic care, even symptomatic improvement became obvious. Kristin was excited to report finally holding in a bowel movement; finally forcing a bowel movement out; and having smaller, less painful bowel movements. Importantly, she was excited about finally having friends. That was a complete life changer for her.

Kristin is now an energetic thirteen-year-old. She excels in school, has many friends, and is even on a competitive dance team. She currently doesn't have any severe bowel problems. Most importantly, Kristin realizes the vital importance of a healthy nervous system, and has brought her family in for Chiropractic care so they can all be healthy.

Dr. Kimberly Koski has been a chiropractor for twelve years, in her hometown of Garson, Ontario. She focuses on family wellness care and strives to live the same lifestyle. Dr. Koski is busy in her practice; as well as in her community. She stays current on what is important in Chiropractic such as research, technique, and philosophy by attending seminars and working towards her ICPA certificate.

Kimberly Koski, DC
Garson Family Chiropractic
1-190 Church St.
Garson, ON P3L-0A1
705-693-0723

Finding Answers and Helping Others

Dr. Russ Derhak

This story has an unlikely beginning, as many great stories do. It starts with a foot, travels to a stomach, and it ends at the pool. This story starts on a beautiful Saturday morning.

I was with my family when I got the call. A mom of a high-level high school athlete needed help. Her son hurt his foot and had a ski meet coming up in the next week. She had heard that Chiropractic was for more than just neck and back issues. So we set off to see if we could help Nathaniel.

During our consultation with them of both, I suggested that we focus on how Nathaniel's nervous system was functioning. I asked, "Have you ever heard that the nervous system is called the master system of the body? If you have heard that, why do you think that is?"

We discussed why all medical textbooks call it The Master System: because the nervous system controls everything in the entire body. I went on to explain that the brain communicates to the rest of the body along wires called *nerves*, and that this system functions like a fuse box. I remember saying, "You know how a fuse box works, right?"

I could see that they were wondering what this had to do with Nathaniel.

I continued. "If something interferes with the fuse, the circuit blows, and nothing on that fuse line functions the way it was designed. So, interference in the body's fuse box (the spine) could result in anything from neck and back pain, to stomach issues, immune system deficiency, concentration issues, and even foot problems like Nathaniel is experiencing."

His mother turned to me with curiosity in her eyes, and hope in her voice. "Do you think you can help my friend's son?"

The honest answer was that I didn't know. But if there was damage to his nervous system, we may be able to help. Now, this is where we leave Nathaniel's story, which in itself is pretty amazing.

This is a story about Nick. It took a few days before we finally got the call. A cautious voice on the other end pleaded, "Do you really think you can help my son?"

Nick struggled with stomach cramps. He had cramps often. He had them hard. In fact, they were so intense that when Nick experienced them, it literally looked like this eleven-year-old boy was giving birth. Can you imagine what this family was experiencing? It took a week before his mother, Janet, called because Nick had again been in the hospital. He had been poked and prodded with every test in the book. The medical doctors tried several different medications, some quite extreme. The doctors were unable to provide any answers. They were baffled.

Could you imagine if your kiddo was going through that? What it must be like to live in constant fear, to experience worry and anxiety, along with the emotional and financial struggle that follows for the whole family? When futures become uncertain, these situations can rip families apart.

Nick was out of school more than he attended. He didn't know if he could play sports. His social life was strained since no one knew what triggered these vicious attacks. Coming to me was their last hope. But this story isn't what Nick overcame. It's really about what he became once his spine was free of subluxations and his nervous system was clear to function as it is meant to function.

After Nick underwent continued Chiropractic care, he went on to play high school football for a team that contended to go to the state tournament. He is an excellent trap shooter. He is so good that he took the state title. He was able to live like a typical kid and hang out with his friends. Things are going so well for him that he's now in high school. He's given up football because he has a passion for swimming. Nick loves being a lifeguard. Now he gets to live an exceptional healthy life, and change lives too.

So, if you are at the end of your rope, if you are exhausted and frustrated, if you've almost given up and are ready to play your last "hope card," it's time to do something new. Take this new path of hope. Find a chiropractor that serves families and focuses on kids. Don't wait. Your family's future can be brighter than ever. Maybe one day, your kiddo's story will be written, just like Nick's.

Oh ... and as for Nathaniel, he consistently improved and the next year he placed high in the state tournament and now skis in college.

Dr. Russ Derhak has a passion for serving kids through the power of Chiropractic. He opened his practice, Inner Light Chiropractic, right out of school in 2006, with the purpose of unleashing boldness in families by focusing on kids. His practice is truly a family affair as his wife, Anna, who has her master's in nutrition, runs the office. They often have their three kiddos around as well, Isabelle, Genevieve, and Lucas.

Russ Derhak, DC
Inner Light Chiropractic, P.A.
4630 Oak Grove Parkway
Brooklyn Park, MN 55443
763-486-3945

"Regular Chiropractic care saves lives,
adds life to your years,
and years to your life."

Gilles A. LaMarche, DC

SECTION FIVE

Immune System
(Infections, Fevers, Failure to Thrive, Asthma)

The Story of Jazzy

Dr. Aixa Goodrich

Since I was a little girl, I always knew I wanted to help others. I dreamed of becoming a doctor someday so that I could see God work his magic through me. From a very young age, I somehow knew that the body was self-healing and self-regulating. What most people would call a miracle is really innate intelligence doing what it does best.

After finding my way to a chiropractor many years ago, I knew that this was the profession I had been looking for my entire life. I am fortunate to have found a profession that cares about its patients, founded on the premise that the body is, in fact, self-developing, self-healing, and self-regulating when free of interference.

I have had the privilege of working with thousands of patients over the last sixteen years. Each was certainly put in my path to teach me something new, to keep my passion burning brightly for removing subluxations, and to deepen my spirituality and allow me to be a better physician and human being.

There are certainly some patients who touch your heart a little deeper than others. For me, one of those people is Jazzy.

Jazzy is a beautiful little girl who was suffering with "unexplained fevers" as described by the allopathic industry. She was five years old when she first came to me. Her parents described how from the time she was born, Jazzy had been getting fevers almost on a weekly basis and was on antibiotics more often than not. They had lost count of the number of times they had to rush her to the Emergency Room (ER) with a fever of 104°F. On any given night, at 3:00 a.m., they'd submerge her in a cold tub to decrease the fever. She was examined by an array of medical specialists who conducted multiple tests. All the pricks, scans, and tests came back negative. Her parents were obviously happy with the negative test results but extremely frustrated from the lack of understanding as to why the fevers kept recurring.

After a thorough history, I examined Jazzy. Her temperature was 103°F that day. She was notably scared, as her experience with doctors had been negative thus far. I found a subluxation in her cervical spine and explained to the parents what the significance of that was. They were happy to finally hear what could potentially be causing the fevers, but also upset that no one, in the last five years, had found said subluxations, or provided any answers.

They consented to have me adjust Jazzy. After her first adjustment, Jazzy took a deep breath as if life had re-entered her body. I told her parents that I would see her again the following day, and that I would continue to see Jazzy daily if necessary. Although her mother did not seem happy with this care plan, as they had driven many miles to get to my office, she reluctantly agreed.

Within a couple hours of her initial adjustment, Jazzy's body temperature returned to normal. I adjusted her every day for one week, with no further signs of a fever—not even a low-grade one. Even after one month, Jazzy has not had another fever.

Jazzy is now ten years old. I humbly report that she has not had a fever or any antibiotics since her first adjustment. Her parents are eternally grateful and I continue to live my purpose of improving lives by educating and empowering people to make better health and life choices.

Aixa Goodrich, DC
Chiropractic Physician
305-271-7447
www.SouthFloridaChiropracticCenter.com

Immune Function and Personality

Dr. Amanda F. Jerviss

Lucy first came to my practice when she was just over two years old. She appeared relatively healthy at the time, but had been a very fussy baby. She also seemed to have a weak immune system. She would get sick easily and would take a long time to get better. Her mom had been a patient in my office for several weeks and wanted to have her daughter's spine checked. Her mother also mentioned that Lucy seemed overly anxious about situations.

When I carefully checked Lucy's spine, I found that her second vertebra in her neck was subluxated, or misaligned, putting pressure on the central nervous system. I gently adjusted her spine and helped clear the nerve interference caused by the subluxation.

Over the next few weeks, her parents reported that she seemed more relaxed and not as shy or jumpy in social situations. When they attended a wedding, Lucy was out on the dance floor with some other children she had just met. Previously, she would have stayed close to her parents and not wanted to be the center of attention. Her parents were ecstatic about the new development. Their child was becoming more confident in who she was and in the world around her. She was not shying away and scared of things that she should be enjoying.

Lucy does not get sick as often as she once did either. Lucy had not been sick for several months, but then developed a fever and a runny nose. Her mother was dreading the next several days. She said, "Everybody in the family is miserable when Lucy is miserable." I adjusted Lucy as soon as they noticed she was fighting something. A couple days later, with relief and joy in her voice, Lucy's mom told me that Lucy was already over being sick. This was a new experience for the family, and a much better experience than they were used to having.

In Lucy's case, Chiropractic changed the course of her life. She went from being a sickly, anxious girl, to a confident, bold, healthy child. She easily makes friends, is outgoing and beautiful. She is not fearful and does not need to take medication on a regular basis.

Lucy's parents had heard that Chiropractic could help boost immunity, but they did not realize Chiropractic would help with a toddler's anxiety levels. They have gratefully enjoyed this happy side-effect.

The fact that the central nervous system controls every cell, tissue, and organ in the body has been beautifully displayed in this child. Hormone and chemical levels are directly controlled by the nervous system. Adjusting the spine affects absolutely every part of the body in ways that science is only beginning to understand.

It brings me inexpressible joy to be a part of Lucy's journey. I love watching her blossom a little more every day into what God intended for her. She is an amazing child.

Amanda F. Jerviss, DC
Jerviss Family Chiropractic
www.VibrantSpine.com

The Power that Made the Body, Heals the Body

Dr. Andrew Moore

Paige started coming to the office four months shy of her eighth birthday, near the end of April. Her mother had been under sporadic Chiropractic care since she was in her teens; and had experienced some great results in my office.

One day, our conversation turned toward whether or not I thought Chiropractic could help Paige. I asked her mother what the concern was or if she was having a health challenge. Paige always had a sore throat and seemed to get sick every six to eight weeks, which would last for one or two weeks at a time. What was even more frustrating for Mom was that this had been ongoing for a few years, and the antibiotics prescribed weren't working and didn't seem to help. Also, Paige was a young, up-and-coming rep hockey player and, after receiving some bumps at the rink, was complaining of a sore neck.

When Paige came in to see me, her neck was so stiff she could hardly turn her head in any direction. Her head was noticeably tilted to the left, and her shoulders were tilting the other way. It didn't take a doctor to see that her body was out of balance. I felt her neck and found a subluxation at the top bone in her cervical spine, called the atlas. Subluxation is the fancy word a chiropractor uses when there is a misalignment in the spine that creates nerve pressure and interference in the body. When there is nerve pressure in the body (especially the neck), muscles get tight, the body becomes imbalanced, and if the affected nerve goes to an organ, it can start to dysfunction.

Her mother was surprised when I asked if Paige was experiencing any breathing difficulties, because I had just found a subluxation in her upper back and those nerves go straight into the lungs and heart. Her mom told me she had recently been diagnosed with asthma.

Paige was a little nervous to get adjusted, until she felt how gentle an adjustment really is. By the end of summertime, Paige hadn't had a sore throat or cold, and her ear aches went away. By the middle of October, not only had she gone two months without missing any school, but she was now completely off her puffers. I think the most satisfying thing Paige told me was she no longer worried when she was on the ice that she might not be able to breathe and had more energy to play in the games.

The body is amazingly powerful, and is naturally programmed to be healthy and well. It is amazing to watch that power come to life when nerve pressure is removed.

Andrew Moore, DC
Moore Chiropractic Centre
275 Trafalgar Road
Oakville, ON, L6J 3H1
905-845-4541
drandrewmooredc@gmail.com
www.moorefamilychiropractic.ca

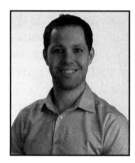

Asthma Relief

Dr. Autumn Gore

"Hey, Dr. Autumn!" called the sweetest little voice from just outside our adjusting space.

As I looked around the corner, Michael's eyes shone brightly, full of LIGHT for the first time since we met just six weeks ago. "How are you brother?" I asked him—a simple question that he had not always been able to completely answer through the coughing and breathlessness that usually consumed him.

His quiet, clear response stopped the high-moving energy around the three adjusting tables in unison. "Today I went to PE and today I didn't have to sit out. Today I played the whole time with all the other kids!"

Tears rolled down my face as he hugged me so hard I was not sure he ever wanted to let go. After a moment, he lifted himself onto the table. As he lie face down, he proclaimed, "I'm a healing machine, y'all!!!"

At five years old, Michael could not remember a time when he hadn't struggled in a fight with asthma. For years, his patient and loving mama woke up with him every night, sometimes several times a night, to give him breathing treatments. Facing the end of medical options, just as so many people find their way into Chiropractic offices around the world, tired of just surviving and fighting, they came in, ready to look beyond treatments and ready to find a solution. Michael was ready to THRIVE.

Within the first week of receiving Chiropractic care and integrating the power released through his adjustments, Michael started to cough less. In two weeks, his mama noticed his sleeping significantly improved and the need for medication decreased. After four weeks, he started sleeping through the night, with no symptoms and no need for medication. He was able to have play dates at friends' houses for the first time because the fear that he would have a crisis was fading away. His sweet, little body was healing.

Michael told us he felt amazing most days, with only a few hard ones scattered in. But in the sixth week, when he was able to play with all the other kids, when he was able to just be himself and play all-out, that's when something deeper healed. Something bigger aligned than just the bones of his spine. The alignment with the healer within, with the innate spark that flows through all of us, making us who we are, reconnected within him and reignited his trust in himSELF.

After his adjustment that day, as he climbed off the table, Michael asked me if I had time to see one other person. Curious, I said sure, and waited at my table as he ran into the reception space and quickly remerged with his sister.

"I want Lola to get adjusted too, Dr. Autumn." Michael stood beside me, beaming with pride as she climbed up and lay face down.

When we experience alignment, we share the spark, whether through our words or just the shift in our presence. Life, light, and joy are infectious. We all have the innate power to HEAL, the courage to GROW, and the potential to THRIVE.

The children in our lives remind us of this every single day.

I serve radical Love and alignment with my husband, Tom, at Cafe of Life, in Dallas, Texas. Together, with the support of a wonderful team of chiropractors, we hold the space with open minds for the entire community to come as they are and be received with open arms. As an Innate Centered office, we know that through the eyes of our creator we all shine in divine perfection. It is our intention to support the journey of everyone we serve in discovering and expressing the best version of themselves. See you on the trail!

Autumn Gore, DC
www.cafeoflifedallaas.com

Ella's Story

Dr. Carolyn Griffin

My daughter was about two years old when we moved into our new home. It was so new that it wasn't even on the map. It was late at night and our son was asleep in his bed.

My husband and I were in the playroom watching a movie and, since our daughter had a fever, I had her sleeping on me so I could keep a close eye on her. I had dealt with fevers before; our son has had 104° to 105°F fevers for four to five days; with regular adjustments, we got him through it. No meds were needed to bring down the fever because that's not how we did things.

It was probably midnight when all of a sudden I felt my daughter's entire body stiffen on top of me. She went completely rigid. I immediately knew something was wrong and screamed at my husband to turn on the lights as I laid her on the floor. It was clear she was having a seizure.

Any parent who has experienced this, knows how horrific it is! I have gone through this with patients before, and managed through with no big deal. But when it's your own child, it's a totally different story! Let's just say, I FREAKED OUT! I'll be the first to admit it. My first reaction was to call 9-1-1. When you see your daughter's eyes roll to the back of her head, not breathing, and lips turning blue … to me, THAT'S an emergency! So I had my husband call.

It took the emergency personnel about twenty minutes to get to our home because they couldn't find it—and thank God for that. During that time, I regained my composure and realized it was a febrile seizure (due to high temperature) and that we could handle this on our own. But all of a sudden we had about seven firemen in our home.

They were adamant about taking her to the hospital and would NOT leave, even though we asked them to on many occasions. So, I finally asked, "What will you do to her if I let you take her to the hospital?"

One fireman responded that they would give her medication to bring down the fever. Well, I knew that wasn't an option for us. So, we again asked them to leave. After making us feel like total crap and horrible parents, they finally left.

I was crying and upset, and Ella was having more seizures. I really wasn't handling this well—it was all very scary!

I called one of my mentors, Dr. Fred Schofield, thinking he would feel sorry for me and calm me down. Well, that's not how it went down ... AT ALL!

He said, "Carolyn, what the F@*k are you doing?"

"What?! Why are you yelling at me?" I was completely rocked back on my heels.

"Carolyn, you're a chiropractor! You're not a mom right now. So, take off your mom hat and put on your Chiropractic hat and take care of your daughter. And do it now!"

At that moment, I felt myself snap out of it and I got to work. I checked Ella and adjusted her. She didn't go to the hospital. She didn't get any Tylenol. She didn't get any medication. And believe me, when it's the middle of the night, it's your two-year-old little girl, and it's all up to you ... yes, I questioned myself. Was I making the right decision for my child? I was afraid. Yes, I was being tested! With the support of my husband, we didn't waiver from our philosophy and we trusted Ella's innate ability to heal!! She experienced more seizures through the night and into the next morning, then her fever broke and it was finally over.

Even though that was one of the worst nights of my life, one that I will always remember, I am thankful for it. It taught me something about myself: to trust the innate ability of people to heal, and to not be afraid! It also made my love, passion, and commitment to Chiropractic even stronger!

Carolyn Griffin, DC
ReVivify
drcarolyngriffin@gmail.com
www.scvchiro.com
www.revivifyme.com

The Ear Infection Plight

Dr. Carla Santin

My daughter Londyn suffered from ear infections since infancy. It seemed that every time she got the sniffles, it would build into a sinus cold, and an ear infection would inevitably follow. This resulted in endless trips to the doctor and emergency room with a very unhappy little girl.

By the time Londyn turned two, she had been on countless rounds of antibiotics and steroid eardrops. It seemed that the infection would clear up and then we would start the cycle all over again.

> We felt helpless. Not only was the constant sickness affecting her demeanor, but her sleep and digestion were also affected.

Londyn was tired and lethargic. She became terrified to go the bathroom because of severe constipation.

Finally, when a head-to-toe rash developed after starting a new antibiotic, we decided she had had enough! At this point, I decided to take Londyn for a consultation with Dr. Carla Santin. Dr. Santin performed a thorough examination and we started a course of adjustments immediately to correct the subluxation in Londyn's upper neck.

The results have been remarkable! Since starting Chiropractic care, Londyn is yet to suffer another ear infection! She made it through the winter with fewer colds and flus, and seemed to bounce back quicker from them. I am no longer anxious about the upcoming cold and flu season. We are getting better sleep in our house and feel like we finally have a happy, healthy little girl to adore.

We may even have a future chiropractor on our hands. Dr.

Santin can't walk into the treatment room without finding Londyn "adjusting" me on the table.

Thank you Chiropractic, for changing our lives!
(Londyn's mother, Diana Wing)

Carla Santin, DC
Santin Chiropractic
44 Algoma St. South
Thunder Bay, ON P7B 3A9
807-344-4606
www.santinchiropractic.com

Barely Surviving to Fully Thriving

Dr. Lindsay McInnis

Imagine your daughter born five weeks early via Cesarean section and weighing only five pounds. Imagine her having to stay in an incubator for eleven days and you leaving the hospital without your firstborn child. Imagine your baby girl projectile vomiting when she finally does come home and losing weight and having to be re-admitted to the hospital just eight weeks later for a major operation: pyloric stenosis.

That was the reality for my parents—and that was my rocky start to life.

I was weak. I was fully vaccinated. I was heavily medicated. And I was unhealthy—a "failure-to-thrive prognosis, with limited social skills, and a lot of work ahead—is what the doctors told my parents.

There absolutely was a lot of work ahead! I was plagued with constant ear infections and given multiple rounds of antibiotics, which made my immune system work overtime and made me susceptible to sickness. I frequently had a cold—blowing and rubbing my nose to the point where the area between my nose and mouth was always red and raw. I had multiple allergies and my family changed their dietary habits to accommodate their young child. The antibiotics for my ear infections didn't always work; so on five separate occasions before I was seven years old, I had operations on my ears to have tubes inserted. My body knew innately that they were not supposed to be there and continued to reject the tubes.

What I remember is the dizzy, headachy feeling of inhaling gas and waking up with blood in my ears. These operations are a lot of stress on a small child, and after each operation my hearing capacity was reduced. "What" and "huh" became my most-used words as I learned to read lips and tried to adjust to my new reality.

When I was in first grade, my mom went back to work full-time—as a Chiropractic assistant. As she was learning about Chiropractic, the chiropractor told her that there was a high chance that the bones in my spine were misaligned due to such a traumatic birth—and that the misalignments created interference in the communication between the brain and the body. When this happens *dis*-ease takes place and the body cannot appropriately adapt to stress, leading to impairment in healing, growth, and function.

Upon hearing this, Mom began to get my younger sister and me checked and adjusted by a chiropractor ... and my whole life changed. My allergies started going away. I was sick less often. And my hearing began to return.

I had dramatic improvements in my health and in my life. I excelled at sports, my grades were remarkable, and I was a very social and energetic kid. From then on, I grew up without drugs and antibiotics, and started allowing my body to heal itself from the inside.

It was that experience that called me to become a chiropractor. This beautiful profession chose me and it was the only thing I ever wanted to be while growing up. I have now been a doctor of Chiropractic for four and a half years, on three different continents, and I am still, and forever will be, humbled by the innate healing power of a body fully connected to itself.

Lindsay McInnis, DC
360 Kiropraktor
Sandvika, Norway
DrLindsayMcInnis@gmail.com
www.360kiropraktor.no

Asthma-Induced Anxiety

Dr. Rachel A. Northern

A mother brought her middle-school-aged son into my office. In her eyes I saw frustration, stress, and worry. She'd heard through people in the community that I might be able to help her son.

Ever since her son was two, he'd had allergy-induced asthma and anxiety. More recently, he'd developed neck pain. The anxiety was severe, especially at night. His mother stayed by his bedside, sometimes for hours, so he could fall asleep. If he woke during the night, he joined his parents in bed so he could fall back to sleep.

I explained to them that I don't treat asthma or anxiety (or neck pain, for that matter). Then I described how we are born to be healthy, and if we aren't healthy, it's usually because of three things. First, we have interference in the master control system of the body (called *subluxations*). Second, we are missing the proper building blocks to heal and repair the body. I said that what I do is remove interference on the nervous system and suggest proper nutrition and supplementation, as needed, to help the body heal naturally.

After evaluating the boy, I found a few subluxations in his neck and upper- to mid-back and very noticeable postural distortions. I recommended a course of Chiropractic care, twice a week for several weeks, and a hair analysis to determine nutritional deficiencies. The boy was excited to start care. I could see hope in his mother's eyes.

Two weeks into Chiropractic care, the boy reported improvement in neck pain and motion, but he still had trouble with anxiety and sleeping by himself.

After two months of Chiropractic care, the son had made

great improvements in his asthma, but he was still having trouble being alone at night and sleeping. He said his thoughts were often negative and he worried that something bad would happen to him.

I asked if he had a history of bad occurrences. He said no. Then I realized I had forgotten to address the third cause of breakdown of health—lack of adaptation to mental stressors. I explained to him how his thoughts create his reality. I visually walked him through ways he could intentionally focus and switch a bad memory or thought into a good one.

When the boy walked into my office after six months of Chiropractic care, he was pain-free, sleeping soundly by himself—even spending the night at friends' houses—and hadn't had to use his inhaler or nebulizer in a month. Plus, he now ran cross-county for his school.

The stress was gone from his mother's eyes. She thanked me for helping her son regain his health and happiness.

This is just one of the many reasons why I love being a chiropractor!

Rachel A. Northern, DC, CACCP
Family Wellness Chiropractor
Johnsburg, IL
www.thedoctorinyou.com

Failing to Thrive

Dr. Ryan French

Cindy was not eating. She was not happy. She was not sleeping. She hated her feeding tube. Cindy was nine months old.

Medically, Cindy was failing to thrive. *Failure to thrive* refers to children whose current weight or rate of growth is much lower than that of other children of similar age and gender.

Since birth, she had a hard time feeding. She wouldn't take to the breast, nor would she take formula from a bottle. They had to resort to a feeding tube because she seemed unable to swallow or even keep any food down. She threw up several times a day. She was on medication to try to keep her from throwing up, and was labeled as suffering from colic as well.

When we met Cindy, she hadn't gained weight for three months. She had the weight of a six-month-old. This is not okay. Her parents were at their wits' end.

When I examined Cindy, I found her to be overly relaxed—almost unable to maintain postural control of her head and upper body. This is highly unusual for a nine-month-old. I found two subluxations in her spine—the ones numbered C1 and T4.

C1, also called the *atlas*, is the main power switch in the body, located at the base of the skull. This area is the one most often damaged during the birth process, especially if forceps or vacuum extractors are utilized. I was told that Cindy had a normal vaginal delivery.

We decided to adjust her atlas using a pediatric toggle headpiece, a special device developed for quickly and accurately correcting the upper cervical region of an infant. There was no distinct sound, nor a reaction from her first adjustment. In fact, Cindy seemed completely indifferent.

I checked her spine every day for one week, and she held her adjustment all week; not needing another adjustment during that time, which was good.

At home, Cindy started to eat. Her parents said she seemed to keep more of her food down. After one week of Chiropractic care, and after months of not gaining weight, Cindy went to the pediatrician for her weekly checkup. Cindy had gained one pound and two ounces in one week!

Within one month, Cindy gained enough weight to be considered average. Her parents were so happy.

We continued to check and adjust Cindy on a wellness basis for another year, until the family moved away. In that time, Cindy hit every normal developmental milestone, which her parents attributed to her Chiropractic care.

In fact, Cindy's grandfather was so happy that his precious granddaughter returned to life and health, that he gifted me with something to help me take care of as many babies as we can—he built two custom-made Chiropractic tables for kids. These tables make kids happy and comfortable in our office, and will continue to bless the lives of many in the decades to come!

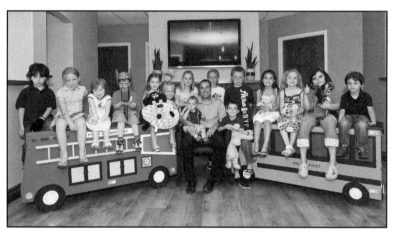

Ryan French, DC
Inside Out Family Chiropractic
27 King Street East
Bolton, ON L7E 1C2
905-951-9911
www.insideoutchiropractic.org

Living through Your Nervous System

Dr. Susanne Morris

Daniel was born one week early and was diagnosed with underdeveloped lungs. Shortly after birth, he was diagnosed with asthma. By the time he was eleven years old, his asthma was so bad that he was using an inhaler eight times a day. He was often admitted in the hospital because of asthma attacks. He was even in the hospital the day before coming into my office.

When he arrived, he complained of headaches, recurrent asthma attacks, and always being tired in the morning. His mother mentioned that he was a mouth breather at night. She also felt he was not developing in size, strength, and coordination as she expected. I explained how we live our lives through our nervous system, and if our nervous system does not work at 100 percent, then our body is unable to function at 100 percent.

Following a thorough consultation and examination, I determined that Daniel suffered from multiple subluxations (spinal areas affecting nervous system function). A care plan was suggested, and both Daniel and his mother agreed to pursue Chiropractic care.

I began working on Daniel, adjusting his spine and removing the areas of nerve disturbance which had prevented his body from working properly. Within one week, Daniel reduced his inhaler dependence to only once per day, and only in gym class. Within five months, his inhaler usage almost became a thing of the past, using it only a few times during the summer.

Can you imagine what Daniel's life would have been like if he had he not discovered Chiropractic care? Time and time again, we see such children in our office and, almost without fail, they regain the health and life they were designed to enjoy.

Over the years, Daniel has been busy going to school, playing football, and snowboarding. Today he is studying science at a local university and still comes in for Chiropractic care.

Susanne Morris, DC
www.calgaryfamilychiro.com

We Vote No Shot

Dr. Victor Benson

In 1996, I was a student clinician at Life University. One week, during church Sunday school, Chris and Melissa came up to me and asked if Chiropractic could help their five-year-old daughter, Brittany. Her tonsils were so enlarged she snored heavily every night. She appeared to be a sickly child, with dark baggy circles under her eyes. She was a surgical candidate to have tonsils and adenoids removed. Chris and Melissa wanted to avoid that, if possible. As we like to say: God doesn't make spare parts.

I asked Chris and Melissa what I ask everyone: "If the lights and TV go out in the living room and you look over and see that the kitchen lights are still on, where do you check for the problem?" Of course, you would check the fuse box.

Your spine is the body's fuse box, with the nerves running out to everything in the body. If there is anything wrong in the body, we want to check the spine.

So, we scheduled an appointment. When Brittany arrived at the clinic, I walked out to the waiting room to say hi while her mom did the intake paperwork. Brittany was grinning ear to ear, so excited to be here.

When it was time to take Brittany back to the exam room, I remember she wanted to hold my hand. It was such a sweet moment. She was smiling and skipping along. And then, all of a sudden, she was crying. I couldn't believe it. I looked around to figure out what she might have seen that would make her cry. I couldn't see anything. So, I stopped and knelt down so I was eye to eye with her and asked her what was wrong.

She said, "I don't want to get a shot."

It took me a second, and then I realized she had always seen me outside of the clinic with regular clothes on; and now she saw me with my doctor's coat and worried she was going to get a shot.

I couldn't help it. I started to laugh and said, "Awww ... don't worry. We don't do that here. We're going to get you better in a different way."

She was happy to hear that.

We found subluxations (vertebral misalignments) in her neck and in upper back, which would disrupt nerve flow to the throat and lung area. Melissa guessed that Brittany had these misalignments because of the stress of the birth process.

We adjusted these areas over a few weeks. We called it "popcorn." It was very gentle and Brittany liked getting adjusted and thought it was fun. Over that time, her tonsils shrunk and the snoring diminished. With better sleep, Brittany's eyes cleared up and she shined with more health and vitality.

And, she didn't get any shots!

Dr. Victor Benson started out as a rocket engineer working for the U.S. Navy before getting the calling to become a chiropractor. He has been a practicing chiropractor since 1997. Alongside his wife, Janet, he has been taking care of the community with a passion for taking care of families and children.

Victor Benson, DC

Benson Chiropractic
116 N. Wisconsin Ave.
Muscoda, WI 53573
608-739-9000
bensonchiro@hotmail.com
bensonchiropracticinmuscoda.com

Blake's Story

Dr. Jake Grinaker

It was a cold, windy January morning as I waited to meet Blake. The only thing breaking the silence in the office was the gentle roar of the furnace as it tried to keep up with the North Dakota winter. As I read the note from Jessica, my CA who had taken the phone call scheduling Blake the day before, I could practically feel Blake's mother's desperation and fatigue.

I soon found out desperation and fatigue were an understatement. The boy carried into the clinic that morning was a grey shell of a three-year old child.

Blake had had so many ear infections, his mom stopped counting at fifty. He had been on a perpetual antibiotic routine for over two years, had two sets of tubes, had his tear ducts probed, and his turbinates cauterized. By this point, his hearing and speech were so delayed he was seeing two different specialists more than three times per week. His mom described their lives as "a living hell" since Blake was nine months. Blake's loving, involved, and well-educated parents had over $100,000 in medical bills with no help, no answers, and no hope.

Blake was spiraling out of control and there was nothing anyone could do about it.

But wait ...

Today was THE DAY Blake found Chiropractic. Blake's loving parents never knew chiropractors worked with children and never dreamed that one could help their son. As I sat back and listened to their story, the struggles and the pains they went through for Blake, my heart sank. After noting every painstaking detail of what Blake had gone through prior to today, all I could say was "I am so sorry." I was sorry this happened to

Blake. I was sorry they had to go through all of the struggle and expense. And I was sorry I wasn't there for Blake thirty months earlier.

I relived Blake's history with his parents and spent time interpreting, discussing, and evaluating all of the episodes, moments, and events leading to this point. I looked up to see tears streaming down their faces. This was the first time in Blake's life someone had listened, someone REALLY cared, and someone had answers.

They had HOPE! We went through a comprehensive Chiropractic examination and found significant upper-cervical subluxations. It was time to get to work ...

Blake's care was intensive and his parents were committed. Following his first adjustment, Blake slept four hours, woke up to eat, and then fell back asleep for twelve more. After eight days of massive sleep and even more drainage, Blake was coming back to life! His speech was improving and his vocabulary exploded. For the first time in his life, he was off all antibiotics and was infection free!

I did not quite realize the extent of the impact our care of Blake had on his family until we received an invitation in the mail to attend a party for Blake. Blake had missed so many holidays and birthday parties while sick and often in the hospital, his parents were throwing him a "Welcome Back to Health" party, and we were the guests of honor. To say Chiropractic care helped with Blake's ear infections would be a drastic understatement. Chiropractic gave three-year-old Blake his life back, and a three-year-old back to his parents.

Jake Grinaker, DC, ACP
Strive Chiropractic
3361 45th St., Ste. #108
Fargo, ND 58104
701-893-4200
www.strivechiropractic.com
facebook.com/StriveChiropractic

"Little" Matty

Dr. Brenda Fairchild

You can never underestimate the power of a Chiropractic adjustment!! Every day I am amazed how many children can be helped by simply having their bodies aligned. To be able to help a family that is scared, frustrated, and has lost hope for their child ever getting better is truly a blessing.

I see kids who have been to the "best of the best" hospitals and physicians in the Northeast, and come back empty-handed, with absolutely no answers or hope of healing. So often, frustrated parents then seek out a pediatric chiropractor, thinking: "Well, what could it hurt? Nothing else is working." Here is a story about little "Matty."

Matty came to my office at three weeks old. He had been in and out of the hospital for "failure to thrive." He was born weighing six pounds; when he arrived at my office, he weighed only three pounds. He was gaunt, his skin was grey to pale-yellow, his tiny eyes were sunken and dark. When he was awake, he was spitting up or trying to poop. He slept almost twenty-two hours a day.

No one could figure out what was happening. The pediatrician told his mother to stop breast-feeding, thinking the baby was allergic to breast milk. They started Matty on formula and medications for possible "silent reflux," then the spit-up turned into projectile vomiting and his weight dropped drastically.

They started him on dairy formula, then switched to soy, to see if the vomiting would calm down. He was slightly better on soy, but then his bowels stopped moving. Mom was at her wits end. She wasn't sleeping, was worried sick about Matty, and wondering what might happen to her little treasure.

When Mom handed me her frail, tiny baby, I was concerned yet honored, and my hands just went to work doing exactly what I know. Matty slept through most of the exam; hardly woke up. His belly was tight and distended; yet over the rest of his body, his skin seemed to just be hanging off of him. While doing the exam, I found misalignments in the upper neck, called the atlas; as well as the sacrum, a bone that lies between the two hips.

More than likely these misalignments happened during the birth process. Mom had a long vaginal labor of over forty-eight hours. I would say OUCH! for both Mom and Matty. Matty had been tucked deep in his mother's pelvis for some time without descending.

Following my examination, I gently adjusted the atlas and the sacrum and worked on the trigger points of his belly—and he pooped immediately! Mom was so happy! They went home that night with some hope. Matty was still on soy at this point and was able to keep more down.

I talked to Mom the next morning, and Matty was more awake than he had been since birth. She was definitely more hopeful.

On the second visit, he was opening is eyes and slightly engaging with me. Vomiting was less. Mom took him off the medicine he had been on. He was pooping more, but very hard and solid, not what a baby should have. We then slowly switched to dairy, and he became more regular.

Following the next few adjustments, Matty showed signs of getting stronger, and there was color returning to his body.

Over the next few weeks, he began to cry—something he had not done before. He started acknowledging all of us, he smiled, and he was able to do some tummy time and hold his head up.

He was gaining weight like a champ and the skin that was hanging off his frail body was starting to fill out.

Today "Little" Matty is over a year old, crawling like crazy, and chunky as can be! He has the most beautiful brown eyes that twinkle, a beautiful sight compared to the eyes we could barely see on the first day.

It is such an honor to help a tiny, fragile baby back to life and to see him THRIVING better than anyone expected.

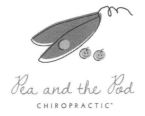

Pea and the Pod
CHIROPRACTIC

Brenda Fairchild, DC, CACCP
Pea and the Pod Chiropractic
One Centurian Dr., Suite 104
Newark, DE 19713
302-455-PEAS (7327)
www.peapodchiro.com
Specialized in Fertility, Women's Health, Pregnancy, and Pediatrics

Immune Function

Dr. Tim Wood and
Dr. Suzie Wood

In my fifteen years of practice, I have discovered that the immune system seems to be the system that is most often easily changed by improving spinal alignment to improve nerve system function. This is especially true in children.

When a child gets adjusted, I expect that they will get sick less often, fight things off quickly, and generally be healthier. As a result, their teachers, coaches, relatives, etc. start to ask what the parents are doing to keep their child so healthy.

One of the most rewarding examples of that positive effect is with my own children. As a family, we are rarely ill. If one of us does get sick, it is usually a one-to-two-day bout and then we are back to 100 percent. In comparison, my children's friends are usually sick for seven days or longer. And, if a family member is ill in our house, most often the others don't get sick. Again, that is not the case for the average family. Once one person is sick, the whole house usually gets it.

Our oldest son, Owen, was always difficult to check and adjust as a child. He would wriggle, stay tense, and just generally be more difficult than the hundreds of other kids I've adjusted. He did not have symptoms, so his adjustments were always preventative, to keep him healthy.

Then, one winter, he had a cough that sounded like croup. I took him down to our basement adjusting table, checked him, and adjusted his spine. He was barking during the process but once he was adjusted, the cough immediately stopped. He looked much better.

None of this surprised me, but it surprised Owen! Maybe he had seen his adjustments as annoying distractions from playing, but that day he recognized how Chiropractic helped his body heal and stop coughing. He lit up. From that moment, he was excited anytime we said the word *adjustment* or went near a Chiropractic table. He even started pretending to adjust my wife and me. Who knows, maybe I will be telling that story at his graduation from Chiropractic College one day. Either way, I am glad Owen finally became one of my best patients to adjust!

Following are two more stories of children's immune systems changing because of Chiropractic adjustments, written by their moms.

~~

This boy came to our office when we practiced in the United Kingdom. I remember he was a sickly looking child. It was my wife, Dr. Suzie, who was taking care of him. We were fresh out of Chiropractic College, but through observing in many offices that saw children, and doing a pediatric fellowship, we knew the potential Chiropractic had to change lives! He was our first pediatric Chiropractic miracle story:

"Who would have thought that a chiropractor could have helped an eighteen-month-old baby? Well, I'm here to tell you that they can. I was admitted to hospital at six months old with bronchitis, and I still wasn't sleeping well. I was regularly waking through the night. After being discharged from hospital, I was put on two types of inhalers, which I apparently hated. It was a constant battle for my mum and dad to give me this medication. In addition, they were getting little sleep; so it was hard on all of us. This continued for at least another eleven months until my mum and dad had an idea. They brought me here and, from then on, my life changed.

"When I first started coming here, I began to sleep and I didn't need my Ventolin inhaler. To this day, I still haven't used it. I am so much happier. I enjoy running, jumping, and have much more fun. I enjoy kicking a ball around, and hopefully one day I'll be a footballer. But for now, I will just enjoy my life, enjoy seeing Dr. Suzie, and being happier.

"Oh, by the way, my mum and dad have noticed the difference and so have my grandparents. I would highly recommend anybody, of any age, to go through Chiropractic treatment. It definitely gives you a new lease on life."

The above was not actually written by T, because he's just about to turn two. But, as his mum and dad, we feel that if he could talk and write, that is what he would say. His life has changed completely, his chest problems are reduced (if not cured), and his sleeping is 100 percent improved. These changes have not only affected T, they've also affected us for the best. We highly recommend Chiropractic treatment for everyone of all ages!

~~

"A year ago, our family sought to find quality Chiropractic care. Reasons for this included neck pain (for our children and me), headaches for our youngest child, and hip pain. We found Mission Chiropractic via Google and picked them because they are a child-friendly clinic.

We attended Dr. Tim's educational meeting and decided to make the commitment to pursue scheduled Chiropractic treatment. As we hoped, our chronic neck, back, and hip pain and headaches went away. Having said that, what came along with this new form of care was remarkable. Having suffered for over ten years with sinusitis, allergies, and other immune issues, I can tell you these symptoms and ailments have all but ended and my overall health has made a dramatic improvement with Chiropractic care.

"As is somewhat expected by all parents, children seem to always be sick. Our children were no different. We eat healthy and are an active family; however it just seemed they could never beat a cold or flu without antibiotics. These mild illnesses would often turn into much worse, such as ear infections, tonsillitis, scarlet fever, allergies, rashes, and croup.

"We cringed when we traveled because we were sure our children would get sick just from setting foot in an airport. I am here to tell you, life does not need to be this way. Our children have missed little to no school due to illness and we have been completely antibiotic free in our house for over one year. We have seen excellent posture improvement as well.

"Chiropractic was the only change we made in our lives; so we are sure that this is a direct result of our newfound care. As I look back at all the lost wages I had from staying home with sick kids, all the medical and herbal purchases made to try to obtain good health, not to mention the damaging antibiotics our children had to ingest, I wish we had found Dr. Tim and his method of treatment much earlier. Chiropractic has allowed a much more balanced and enjoyable life for my family and me. We would like to thank Dr. Tim and his staff at Mission Family Chiropractic."

Tim Wood, DC and Suzie Wood, DC
Mission Family Chiropractic
#10 – 3818 Gordon Dr.
Kelowna, BC V1W 4V1
250-712-0900
www.missionchiropractic.ca
info@missionchiropractic.ca

Little Ali—from Sickness to Thriving

Dr. Kareen Oosterhart

This is Allison. She is currently four years old and a bundle of energy and curiosity. I always look forward to my weekly visits with Ali, her mom (Kim) and sister (Mackenzie). Ali loves her adjustments so much that we have to keep track of who goes first from one visit to the next to make sure she shares with her sister.

Kim said Ali's life started well. Kim had a healthy pregnancy, had no complications during birth, and Ali was the healthy baby they expected. As a child, Kim had a history of ear infections; and in Ali's first six months, she had them as well. Ali was treated with antibiotics, but as soon as she was off of them her fevers would spike again. The doctors assumed it was her ears and would place her on antibiotics again—only for longer periods.

The cycle repeated.

One weekend, Ali became very ill. Her fever spiked to 105°F, so her parents gave her ibuprofen to bring down the fever. By the time they decided to take her to the hospital, Ali was shaking so much the nurses said she was having convulsions. Ali was going into septic shock. Her body was beginning to shut down because of the infection and her body was having trouble fighting it.

This was not a typical ear infection. The doctors ran numerous tests on Ali to find the cause. They also pumped her full of antibiotics and fluids because she was now dehydrated. One of the things they checked for was leukemia because her white-blood cells were so high. Fortunately these tests came back negative. All they found was a severe urinary tract infection; so the course of treatment was more antibiotics.

When Ali was stable, they sent her home. Fortunately for Ali and her family, their family medical doctor was not satisfied with the hospital's findings. He thought there had to be a reason besides a urinary tract infection for Ali to have become so ill. So he scheduled an appointment with a pediatric urologist to determine the cause of Ali's continuous infections. Their family doctor felt that it might be a reflux problem within the urinary tract, meaning that her urine was backing up and causing the infections.

The pediatric urologist ran a voided cyst urethrogram (VCUG) on Ali. They placed a catheter in her little body and ran iodine through the catheter, into her urethra, and up to her kidneys to see if the system was working properly. They found that all of her "parts" were there, but the sphincter between the urethra and the kidneys was not closing; thus allowing the urine to flow back into the kidneys.

The only option given to her parents was to keep Ali on antibiotics so her kidneys did not become so infected, otherwise they could discontinue working. The urologist told Kim that the sphincter problem was probably due to nerve damage.

They had no way of knowing for certain and no way to fix it. The only way to help Ali was to keep her kidneys free of infection to help assure that Ali would be less likely to need dialysis when she was older. (Most people with this problem are on dialysis by the age of thirty if they do not remain on medication.) He also told Kim that Ali would probably always have bed accidents, and might not be able to be potty trained because of the nerve damage to her urinary system.

Kim was not willing to accept the idea that her child's body could not heal. She began to research what would help. She felt that if it was a nerve problem, the nerves needed to be stimulated in some way. That is what brought Ali to our office a few weeks before her first birthday. We began checking Ali for subluxations (nerve interference) and found that her sacrum was not moving properly and that there was a problem with her C1 (first cervical vertebra) in her neck. The nerves that exit at the sacrum feed the urinary system and can be related to problems with bedwetting and the urinary tract when interfered with. C1 subluxations affect everything from hormones to the immune system.

Ali continued taking antibiotics and received VCUG testing every six months until she was two, then again one year later. Between the ages of two and two-and-a-half, her mother felt Ali was getting better because by then Ali was potty-trained. At three, it was discovered that Ali's urethra sphincter was fully functioning. It was at this time that Ali was weaned off of the antibiotics.

Ali was headed down a life of continued medications that would have affected not only her bowels and her immune system, but her entire life. Had it not been for a concerned physician and a determined mother, Ali's future would have had a different outcome. Today, her little body is functioning the way God designed it to function, with her nervous system intact and communicating to every system in her body.

Ask Ali and her mom how important and life-changing an adjustment can be—I am sure they would love to tell you.

Kareen Oosterhart, DC
Village Chiropractic Wellness Center, P.L.C.
798 W. Mile Rd.
Kalkaska, MI 49646
231-258-4023
www.village-chiropractic.com

Sweet Magnolia

Dr. Erin Stark Calaway

On the afternoon of April 30, 2015, I walked into my pediatric adjusting room and was greeted by the most cheerful, sweet, smiling girl. Little did I know that Magnolia was actually having a lot of ear pain and loss of hearing from suffering ear infection after ear infection.

After several rounds of antibiotics and being told her daughter needed tubes, Magnolia's mother knew there had to be another option. She searched a mom's group on Facebook, asked for a chiropractor, and I was recommended. Magnolia's mother told me I was her last resort, and that she was very skeptical.

It was imperative I educate this mother and child, to make them both comfortable with me, and to let them know they were in very good, loving, healing hands. I explained Chiropractic, the spine, the nervous system, and their effects on the entire body and all of our systems. I needed both of them to understand how Chiropractic adjustments of Magnolia's spine would help her nervous system function as it should. With a properly functioning nervous system, the possibility of healing would be greatly enhanced. And yes, the ears do receive nerve supply, and the return of full nerve supply could solve Magnolia's issues, even restore her hearing. (Most people do not know that the first documented Chiropractic adjustment performed by Daniel David Palmer on a deaf janitor, named Harvey Lillard, on September 18, 1895, resulted in Harvey regaining his hearing.)

After my examination, I knew Magnolia needed a really powerful adjustment. So, that's exactly what I did! I turned this little girl's power on in the most amazing way!! Her testimonial says it all:

"Our family found Chiropractic due to our daughter, Magnolia, having trouble hearing. We first went to her pediatrician when we noticed her frequently asking 'What?' Her pediatrician cleaned the wax from her ears and eventually referred us to an Ear, Nose, and Throat specialist when we saw no improvement. Magnolia's ENT tested her hearing and found she was lacking about 30 decibels of hearing, the equivalent of living with earplugs. He prescribed an over-the-counter allergy medication and told us that if her hearing was not improved within six weeks, she would need tubes.

That's when we decided to try Chiropractic as a last-ditch effort to avoid sedation and surgery for our sweet four-year-old. We were so lucky to find Dr. Erin. During Magnolia's first adjustment, she looked up at Dr. Erin and told her she loved her!

We were nervous to have her adjusted, but in the car on the way home after her first appointment, Magnolia said that everything was louder! We were excited, but remained skeptical.

After six adjustments with Dr. Erin, we returned to the ENT. Magnolia's audiology test came back 100 percent! She now has monthly adjustments with Dr. Erin, and has had no issues with her hearing whatsoever. We are thrilled with the results we have seen with Chiropractic care and are enthusiastic to spread the word of its benefits.

Thanks Dr. Erin!"

Erin Stark Calaway, DC
APEX Wellness Center
6009 Belt Line Rd., Suite 110
Dallas, TX 75254
972-392-9402
www.apexwellnesscenter.com

SECTION SIX

Behavioral, Neurological, and Other Diagnoses

Brain Function Normalized

Dr. Amy Gatlin

On May 28, 2015, seven-year-old Madelyn was brought into the office by her mother. Her mother reported that Madelyn has been experiencing involuntary eye rolling while blinking, which began about six weeks ago. It occurs with no apparent trigger or pattern. At first, it was very frequent, occurring several times per minute, but it had now decreased to a couple of times per day.

Madelyn's mother reported that she took her daughter to see a neurologist, who ordered an EEG. The EEG was inconclusive, but did show signs of seizures. The neurologist suggested medication to manage the episodes. However, before beginning medication, the mother was seeking Chiropractic care for Madelyn.

I examined Madelyn's spine, following the Gonstead Chiropractic technique protocol. At this visit, she responded well to instructions and was comfortable in my office, having been here before with her father and brother. Abnormal skin surface temperature differentials obtained with a Gonstead nervoscope were noted at the upper cervical, T6, T12, and second sacral tubercle vertebral segments. Static palpation of the spine revealed tenderness and localized edema at S2 and the upper cervical area, specifically C1. Motion palpation demonstrated marked reduced motion at the C1 and S2 (upper and lower parts of the spine).

I discussed these finding with her mother and explained that Chiropractic care sought to relieve the pressure on the nervous system to allow the brain to fully communicate with the body to restore normal function. Madelyn seemed to be experiencing abnormal functioning in the brain, as evidenced by the inconclusive EEG. I further explained that recent studies have shown Chiropractic adjustments have improved the efficiency of the brain function.

We agreed to begin care. I gently adjusted Madelyn at the C1 and S2 segments. Madelyn tolerated the adjustment well, with no problem. I asked the mother to return with Madelyn for a follow-up appointment the next week.

At the second visit, a week later, the mother reported a decrease in the involuntary eye movements but also added, "The frequency was reducing anyway." The real test would be the results of the second EEG, which was scheduled in four days.

I again adjusted C1 and S2, and asked her to return in two weeks, after the second EEG study and allowing more healing time. When they returned on June 19, 2015, the mother reported there had been no involuntary eye movements since the last adjustment and the second EEG was completely normal. Furthermore, the EEG was run for a longer period of time than the first and showed no abnormality whatsoever.

I now see Madelyn once per month. By the end of the month, Madelyn experiences one episode of involuntary eye movement. However, after she receives her Chiropractic adjustment, the involuntary eye movement resolves. Mom and I are convinced the Chiropractic adjustment is the effective factor in solving the involuntary eye movement, and in restoring the normal function of the brain, as demonstrated by the EEG.

Amy Gatlin, DC
Thornton Chiropractic Life Center, PA
2404 Dr. Martin Luther King, Jr. Blvd.
New Bern, NC 28562
252-638-8121

Blessings upon Blessings

Dr. April Lee

All three of my children have been under Chiropractic care since they were babies. Chiropractic care has helped us navigate colic, ear infections, digestive issues; and has all but eliminated the need for sick visits to our pediatrician. I have always been pro-Chiropractic care, but it was not until my third child, Benny, was born that I felt as if the light went on and I truly realized the power of spinal alignment and natural healing.

Benny was born with Down syndrome and a congenital heart condition that is commonly associated with Down syndrome.

As we watched him struggle in his first three months leading up to open-heart surgery, Chiropractic care was the furthest thing from my mind.

When we came home from the hospital after his first surgery, Ben's heart was repaired, but there had been complications during the procedure that resulted in Ben having to go on a totally fat-free diet, indefinitely. I was still reeling from the surgery, the complications, new around-the-clock medications, and researching everything I could think of to help my son heal, when our family chiropractor, Dr. Lee, reached out to me to suggest giving Ben a fish oil supplement to help with the healing process.

She had my attention. I made an appointment for Ben with the intention of only discussing the fish oil to find out if I could give him the fish oil when he had orders for a no-fat diet. During that appointment, Dr. Lee offered to research and verify whether or not fish oil would be safe with Ben's specific complications. As we discussed his case further, I explained that I was concerned about his breathing, especially at night, because of a specific position he would put his head in when I lay him down flat in a bed. We had been to his cardiologist and pulmonologist and neither had an explanation or seemed concerned.

Dr. Lee and I also discussed Ben's severe reflux and my concerns that he was maxed out on all of the medications that were "safe" for pediatric patients, and he was still having significant issues.

After Dr. Lee examined Ben, she noted an issue with Ben's atlas and occiput (top bone of the spine and skull) and asked if she could adjust him. She did so while holding him in her arms. She also felt she could help with his reflux.

To make a long story short, Ben never went into the strange position with his head in bed again; and after regular adjustments, he was weaned totally off of his reflux medications. Dr. Lee has helped Ben in numerous ways, from sinus issues, ear infections, and gently molding his head as he grew.

She again stepped in when scar tissue started to develop at his surgical site. He developed scar tissue on his sternum that resembled a shark fin that was interfering with him lying on his stomach at a very critical time in his gross motor development. Again, I took him to every specialist and after exams and X-rays, was told that it was one of the sternotomy wires that was not lying flat. It could not be fixed unless he needed open heart again in the future. I was told it was something we would have to deal with.

I sought out Dr. Lee again. She researched and suggested a modified type of acupuncture that was shown to be successful in treating scar tissue. And the rest is history.

The scar tissue shrank over time to the point that you have to really feel Ben's sternum to know where the scar build-up was. Ben is now three, and nonverbal. Because he has been going to Dr. Lee's office since he was just a few months old, he is very comfortable receiving adjustments. He has days when he is not feeling cooperative about lying on the table, but Dr. Lee allows him to find a spot, sometimes in my arms, sometimes on the table, sometimes on the floor, and adjusts him where he is comfortable. He sometimes turns around to look at her hands, but then allows her to continue. And when we leave, he has progressed to hugs and a kiss, which is a very big deal to get from Ben.

Dr. Lee is so much more than our "back pain" chiropractor. She is an integral part of our wellness team and we are blessed to know her.

April Lee, DC
Bluewater Chiropractic Wellness Center
4400 Hwy 20 E., Ste. 207
Niceville, FL 32578
www.BluewaterChiropractic.com
850-897-1177

A Classic Case of Tourette's

Dr. Dan DeLuca

The following events occurred during my Chiropractic career when I felt there was so much negativity directed at our profession in the media and the public eye that I started to question why I had chosen to become a chiropractor in the first place. Thankfully this event opened my eyes to the full potential of Chiropractic, and I never questioned my career choice again.

The profession was relatively new to Glasgow, Scotland; and being one of only a handful of Chiropractors in the city, my practice was busy. But I soon fell into the trap of only treating patients for pain. Once they felt better, they left.

It was not long before I started to feel I was doing a disservice to my patients by not providing a wellness-based type of care, the type of care I was trained to deliver; to take care of the person, not the symptom. It was not a fulfilling way to practice and I was looking for a sign that would lead me back to a wellness-based form of practice that didn't just get people out of pain but actually allowed the body to heal itself and keep them healthy.

The sign came to me like a slap in the face.

It was momentarily quiet in my office one day when a lady walked in with just a hint of impatience and a slight look of distress on her face. Mary entered the waiting room and approached my staff. What came next really threw me for a moment. I didn't know how to respond to her request. With the most inquisitive look, she asked, "Can you treat Tourette's? I have a seven-year-old girl with it." I paused for a second, trying to process her question, and before I could answer, she continued, "Because I was on the Internet and I read about a chiropractor who helped a child with Tourette's in California."

I paused again, tilted my head to one side, and thought to myself, *Well, if it's been done before, why not again?* What you need to understand is that anything you do as a chiropractor has to somehow relate to the spine, nerves, or a joint in order to treat it. This was not apparent to me in this case, at least not yet.

I asked Mary where she had gotten the diagnosis for her daughter. She replied that she had been to several specialist neurologists over the course of three years and they all said the same thing: 'She'll just have to live with it.' "I've tried everything except this," she said.

I could sense deep desperation as those words left her mouth, desperation only a mother would have as she imagined her daughter's future slip away from her. Being a recent new parent myself, I couldn't refuse Mary the hope that we might be able to do something for her daughter; so I offered the following, "If I can find something to treat in her spine, then I can treat her for that. If there is some relationship between her spinal issues and her Tourette's, then perhaps there is a chance we can help her." I did not have the confidence to say anything more concrete. And I further offered, "I will not charge you for the treatment unless we see an improvement."

The next day, Mary arrived with her daughter, Angela. Angela was a bright, cheerful lass, but she could not sit still in class and was falling behind in her education. When I entered the exam room, Angela was twitching, chirping uncontrollably, and shrugging her shoulders with each tic. She had classic Tourette's syndrome. Mary explained that it began three years prior, with no previous symptoms.

I examined Angela's spine. She had the most subluxated neck I had seen on any person under the age of twenty. I immediately asked Mary when Angela had injured her neck. After a long pause, she replied, "Well, she did fall off a bunk bed onto her head."

"When?" I asked.

"About three or four years ago."

Bells were going off in my head! "Was this just before the Tourette's symptoms started?"

"You know, I think you are right!" she exclaimed. "It was a few months before, but I never made the connection."

"I will treat Angela for her neck issues," I said, "BUT, her Tourette's may get worse, better, or it may not change at all. I don't want to see the last possibility. If her neck issues are related to her condition, then her symptoms will change; if not, then they will not change." I told Mary not to worry if the symptoms worsened immediately after the treatment because that would be a good sign that the adjustments were having an effect.

Sure enough, Angela started having rapid tics and more chirping and shoulder shrugging right after her first adjustment. I told Mary they would settle down overnight and Angela should have a good sleep."

That night, Angela slept the longest her mother could remember.

I got a call the next day from Mary, around noon. She was excited and told me, Angela hadn't had a tic all morning!

Over the course of the next several weeks, she reacted the same way to her treatment. After a few months, Angela was going more than a week without a tic. At age eleven, when I last saw Angela before I moved back to Canada, she was going four months without a tic, was a star student, and played soccer for a local club. Even at four months apart, her symptoms would only show up as the mildest tic for a day or two before her appointment. When I left Scotland in 2013, the hardest moment I had was saying good-bye to Angela and her family, because they truly opened my eyes to what I believe many chiropractors, and many in the general public never see: the miracles of this profession.

Never underestimate, as I did, what Chiropractic can do for you and your family.

Dan DeLuca, DC
Allandale Chiropractic
27 Gowan St., Barrie, ON L4N 2N9
705-794-5859 (Cell)
705-726-9292 (Office)

The Path from Nonverbal to ...

Dr. Denise Scott

I met Maria through a mutual friend at a networking event. Maria asked if I cared for children in my office. I told her yes and she shared that she had a six-year-old son with autism. She had read that Chiropractic could help with some of the sensory-processing problems that are common for autistic children.

I gave her my business card and several months later they began care in my office. Isaiah was nonverbal and hyperactive. We began weekly care; and after about three months, I asked Maria if there was any difference in his behavior. Maria told me that Isaiah was much calmer and if they missed their appointments they could definitely tell.

One day, she told me she had a surprise. She began to sing "Old MacDonald" and Isaiah joined in on the "E I E I O" part of the song. I was so excited and overjoyed that tears welled up in my eyes.

When I met Maria, I was new in practice and had the desire to have a family wellness practice with a lot of children. I knew in my heart that Chiropractic could help her son and make a difference in the life of her family, but I did not have the actual proof. I kept thinking: all I need is one opportunity that will change things in my practice for the better.

Maria and Isaiah have been with me for over a year and are like family to me. Maria always offers encouragement to me as an entrepreneur and Isaiah gives me all the hugs I need.

I am thankful for the opportunity to serve such a wonderful family and I hope this story is a breath of fresh air for someone in a similar situation. I didn't feel like I had done much but I realized that a little bit goes a long way.

I was reminded of the quote from Dr. B. J. Palmer, the developer of Chiropractic:

"You never know how far-reaching something you think, say or do today, will affect the lives of millions tomorrow."

The next time I meet a mother of a child with a sensory-processing disorder or a mother wanting to give her child the best chance at living a healthy life, I will be able to say with confidence that when your child's nervous system is free of interference, it can overcome whatever challenge he or she has been labeled with.

Denise Scott, DC
Circle of Healing Chiropractic
215 Dalton Drive
Suite C4 Desoto, Texas 75115
214-628-1952
www.circleofhealingchiro.com

Concentration, Emotion, and Behavior

Dr. Mark Kasiban

I remember meeting Seth and his parents, when Seth was about three and half years old. His mother brought him in because he was having behavioral issues. They were told that their little boy might have Attention Deficit Hyperactivity Disorder (ADHD) and he was also being observed for possible autism.

Even though my Chiropractic assistant told me that Seth was throwing books all over the reception area, I was calm and yet excited to meet the little guy. I only hoped he'd let me examine his spine.

When I started to talk and interact with Seth, I didn't see a "problem child." I was able to have fun with him and establish wonderful rapport. He was well-behaved during our first meeting. I thought, "He's just a kid with lots of energy" and I began to doubt the label that was being given to him.

After examining Seth, I found vertebral subluxations in his spine, particularly in the cervical (neck) area. I explained to his parents the effects of subluxations to the nervous system and how they could influence concentration, emotion, behavior, and so much more.

After his first adjustment, his mother told me that Seth had the best sleep he'd had in a while. He was calmer. Seth's grandparents and teacher also commented on how much calmer he was. His parents were so happy. Seth gave me a big hug and high-five before he left one of his first visits. What a sweet kid!

I continued to see and adjust the entire family (including Seth's little sister) for approximately two years before they moved to the United States. Seth continued to improve and has grown to be a healthy, young boy with a passion for music.

Following their last visit to my office, this wonderful family gave me a card thanking me for helping them. This is what was written in it: "Thank you for loving our kiddos. You saw Seth for who he could be. It brought us hope when we'd run out."

I remember Seth so well because he was one of my first clients where I saw what many might consider a Chiropractic miracle, outside of helping people with back pain and neck pain. It made me realize the true power of Chiropractic and how a healthy nervous system can change people's overall health and lives.

I think about how many families in this wonderful world who have no idea how Chiropractic can help them. This thought drives me each day to share the Chiropractic message.

Mark Kasiban, DC
Ajax Family Chiropractic
145 Kingston Road East, Unit 13
Ajax, Ontario, Canada L1S 7J4
905-426-4116
drmark@kasibanchiropractic.com
www.ajaxfamilychiro.com

Amber's Song

Dr. Darrin Groleau

Lucy had been a patient of mine for many years and had experienced great success through Chiropractic. She understood the principle that any subluxation (interference in her nervous system) automatically creates a state of decreased function in the body, and that her Chiropractic adjustments didn't treat any symptoms or conditions, but instead removed and controlled those subluxations thereby allowing her body to heal and function better.

During one of her regular appointments, she asked if I would be willing to help her four-year-old granddaughter, Amber. I came to learn that Amber had been a happy, healthy child who had been growing and developing normally until just before her second birthday when she received her eighteen-month vaccinations. It was at this time that Amber "mysteriously" stopped all verbal communication, became totally introverted, non-functioning, and almost completely unresponsive.

Now, at the age of four, she was labeled severely autistic and to such a degree that Lucy's daughter and son-in-law (Amber's parents) were told by the medical profession that Amber would never be able to attend school and they should be prepared to be Amber's caregiver for the extent of her lifetime.

Of course, I agreed to help in any way that I could.

Following a thorough Chiropractic examination, it was determined that Amber did indeed have multiple subluxations throughout her nervous system; so I began adjusting her as frequently as I could. You see, Amber and her parents lived two and a half hours from my office; so Lucy would make the five-hour round trip, picking Amber up in the morning, bring her to me for her adjustment, and then drive her home that same day. We continued this routine as best we could for a number of weeks with little to no observable changes, but we all knew that healing takes time and none of us were willing to give up on little Amber.

Then came that wonderful day none of us will ever forget. I was busy adjusting patients when I heard beautiful singing coming from our reception area.

Curious to know who was serenading the office, I went to investigate and found this precious little girl, who hadn't spoken a single word in over two years, not only talking—she was singing. With tears streaming down her face, Lucy informed me that since her last adjustment, Amber had just started to sing and had not stopped. I guess that she had to make up for all the lost time of not being able to express herself.

From that point forward, Amber's healing progressed at a staggering rate. So much so, that during the following summer, her parents decided to have her re-evaluated.

Not only did Amber test high enough that she was going to be able to attend school in September, but she was going to be placed in a normal class as her new test results actually graded her as above average with absolutely no signs of autism whatsoever.

In every way, Amber was once again a "normal" child and the medical profession described her healing as nothing short of miraculous.

I shudder to think what the future would have held for this little angel had her family simply accepted Amber's condition as permanent. Thank goodness Lucy insisted that there was still hope and that Chiropractic was the answer. Thank goodness Lucy knew better.

Over my twenty years as a health care professional, I have had the honor of helping tens of thousands of people achieve better health and a better quality of life by recognizing the limitless potential of the human body. Through the aid of Chiropractic, this limitless potential available to everyone is allowed to be expressed. During this time, I have also been privileged to see many so-called miracles that have left an indelible impression on me as both a doctor and as a person.

Amber's journey and ultimate recovery brought tears of joy to my eyes, and will forever remain in my heart.

DR. DARRIN GROLEAU is a family chiropractor practicing in Bolton, Ontario. Together with his amazing team of like-minded doctors of Chiropractic and support staff, he has helped build one of the largest family wellness centers in the country.

Dr. Darrin received his doctorate in 1994 from the Palmer College of Chiropractic located in Davenport, Iowa, following the completion of his Bachelor of Science degree in the field of Kinesiology (the scientific study of the human body) from the University of Waterloo in Waterloo, Ontario.

He is blessed with a wonderful family, comprised of his incredible wife, best friend and soul mate, Lori; along with their amazing children, Daniel and Caitlyn.

Darrin Groleau, DC
Inside Out Family Chiropractic
27 King Street East
Bolton, Ontario, Canada L7E 1C2
905-951-9911
www.drdgroleau@gmail.com

Enhanced Quality of Life

Dr. Maggie Hunsicker

In July 2009, Amanda was twelve years old when she was diagnosed with Rett Syndrome through a genetic blood test. They thought she might live to the age of thirteen or fourteen, but certainly not into adulthood.

Her mother explained that the main areas of concern for girls with Rett Syndrome are cardiac development of a long QT wave and ventricular fibrillation. She stated: "Amanda does not have either of these conditions at this present time."

Individuals with this condition also deal with low gastro-intestinal motility and have difficulty maintaining weight. Amanda had years of problems with weight loss, and now she was dealing with weight gain. She related having to struggle to chew and experiencing swallowing issues during times of stress. On bad days, she does not feed herself, and drinks from straws to minimize the swallowing of air.

Another main concern is mobility. Amanda had multiple experiences with needing to use a wheelchair or walker because of weakness and lack of coordination. She also experienced many falls due to clumsiness.

Many children with Rett Syndrome never speak, use their hands, or are able to walk. Amanda is at risk of losing these skills, and her neurologist is certain that she will lose mobility and require full-time care at some point in the next couple of years.

Here is a rendering submitted to our office by Amanda's mother: "We went to see Dr. Maggie Hunsicker thinking Amanda was having great pain, possibly in her upper back and head. After a thorough examination with Dr. Maggie, it became apparent the intense pain was from the lower back.

Following all of the radiographs back to 2009, we see the injury occurred in January 2014 when Amanda had a twisting fall resulting in a broken first metatarsal. Since she does not communicate pain, the back injury was not suspected.

"Dr. Maggie explained in great detail how her nervous system is under a tremendous amount of stress due to the structural changes in her spine. She also shared that the chemical, physical, and emotional stressors of her everyday lifestyle can play a role in her overall quality of life. Children with Rett Syndrome are likely to have scoliosis. We were told Amanda had this condition when she was very young.

"Dr. Maggie compared X-rays to show us the progression and changes of her spinal curvature. It was great to actually be told what was going on inside; it all made sense! Amanda has been seen weekly by Dr. Maggie for sixteen weeks. Dr. Maggie has been gently adjusting Amanda, has helped us clean up her gut by testing her food sensitivities, and recommending a wellness plan and proper supplementation. Amanda has made amazing and unexpected recovery in several areas of concern since we first saw Dr. Maggie in May 2015. Amanda visited her neurologist at the beginning of September 2015 for a routine checkup. After consistent Chiropractic care, her height measurements show that she has gained two inches just from improvement in her posture. She has shown improvement in useful speech and the ability to communicate her needs, her physical mobility, sleep, posture, gut motility, and digestion. Amanda's pain levels have significantly decreased. She also has a much better ability to organize her thoughts to process the proper response.

"She has been able to discontinue many of the longtime medications she's needed to improve sleep, decrease pain, and improve physical mobility. It really has been a miraculous experience. Amanda just celebrated her twentieth birthday, and every week we see new improvements. Chiropractic care has given us hope and a sense of peace. It has truly been a blessing to finally find what we've been looking for!"

It is good that Amanda's mother suspected back pain, prompting her to bring Amanda to see us. The care provided in this short period has significantly enhanced Amanda's life.

What if Amanda's mother had known about the benefits of Chiropractic care earlier? What if all parents discovered the value of having their children checked by a chiropractor early on in their life? Chiropractic is not about treating a symptom; it's about allowing the human body to function as it should, without interference.

Who do you know who would benefit from Chiropractic care?

Dr. Maggie received her certification in Chiropractic Pediatrics with the International Chiropractic Pediatric Association and is also Webster Technique Certified. She has a strong affection for pregnancy and pediatric patients but believes that Chiropractic care is essential for all ages. As a fourth-generation graduate from Palmer College of Chiropractic, Dr. Maggie is dedicated to encourage, educate, and inspire individuals to incorporate Chiropractic care into their lifestyle.

Maggie Hunsicker, DC
www.drmaggieh.com

Noah

Dr. Michael Staffen

Noah seemed like every other nine-year-old boy when he was in my office, but his mom explained that it was a different story when he was at school. Noah had been diagnosed with ADHD and was a terror at school. He didn't listen, was always getting in trouble, didn't concentrate, and was a frequent fixture in the principal's office.

The doctors were pushing hard for Noah's mom to put him on medication to control him, and the school was very much behind the doctors' decision. However, a family friend suggested that maybe Noah should seek some help at my office. This friend was a patient in our clinic and knew that we have had some success with kids with ADHD.

Noah's mom had nothing to lose, as she was at her wits' end. During the case history, she explained that he was never a good sleeper, much like herself, and that he had problems with chronic recurrent ear infections—having multiple rounds of antibiotics as well as six surgeries for tubes in his ears—with not much change.

However, the ADHD was the biggest problem! A physical examination revealed spinal subluxations in the cervical (neck), thoracic (upper back), and lumbar (lower back) regions. I explained that subluxations affect how messages from the brain travel down the spinal cord and back up to the brain. These subluxations will be affecting Noah's health and possibly showing up as ADHD. We started on a course of treatment of twice per week.

After a few weeks, we began to see some changes with Noah. My staff remarked that Noah was such a nice boy, he would walk behind the reception desk and give each of them a hug after his treatment.

A few weeks after, Noah's mom told me, with a smile, that the secretaries at the school office had stopped her in the hall and asked her what medication she had put Noah on because he was a changed boy. She proudly explained that there was no medication, just Chiropractic care!

As the weeks of treatment continued, one day Noah's mom said, "Noah, tell Dr. Staffen what happened at school today."

Not knowing what to expect, I braced myself for bad news; however, I was delighted to hear that he had been awarded Student of the Month! Seeing Noah's great results, his mom soon became a patient and she too saw the benefits of Chiropractic care for her heartburn and long-term sleeping problems.

Another good surprise came near the end of school, when Noah came in one day with a medal around his neck. Smiling ear to ear, he said, "Dr. Mike, I got the Most-Improved Student of the Year!"

His mother's eyes watered with joy as she told me that the doctors had told her that Noah would never amount to much and was destined to be in jail unless she put him on medication. She was overjoyed that Noah and her health had improved so much over the past year.

Michael Staffen, DC
New Sudbury Chiropractic & Wellness
1100 Lasalle Blvd.
Sudbury, Ontario, Canada P3A 1X9
705-521-1100
drmikestaffen@sympatico.ca

The Fog has Lifted

Dr. Ryan French

Many of us believe that if we drink water, eat right, and get adequate exercise we'll be healthy. All good advice, but what happens when things don't go according to plan? Tanner's world drastically changed in 2000 when he experienced his first of what would become thousands and thousands of seizures.

His mother started researching, and their journey of hope took them in many directions. From numerous hospitals, general practitioners, neurologists, naturopaths, homeopaths, a shiatsu master, and the Ketogenic Diet Clinic at the Hospital for Sick Children in Toronto. Through trial they discovered that Tanner is allergic to anticonvulsant drugs and the medical model wasn't providing answers or hope.

Tanner and his mother, Cynthia, embarked on a three-and-a-half-year culinary challenge with the Ketogenic Diet Clinic. Seizure activity did, indeed, decrease but what emerged was a four-week seizure cycle. For one week, once a month, the seizure activity would return and build gradually, peaking in the middle of the week, with as many as four to six seizures that night and then falling off again toward the end of the week. Then a "recovery" week marked with insomnia, delayed response time, slowed speech, short-term memory loss, and general brain fog—only to repeat the pattern in the next two weeks, over and over again. Cynthia began to wonder if this was as good as it was going to get.

Finally they were introduced to a chiropractor who embraced a natural approach to healing and didn't only offer care but empowered them through knowledge. After attending an informational evening, they left with a better understanding of how the brain and body communicate and what can happen when there is interference; interference that you may or may not even know is there. This interference, called *vertebral subluxation*, prevents the signals traveling along your spinal cord from getting to their destination: your systems, organs, and cells. What a simple, yet powerful message!

After noticing that one of Tanner's shoulders was significantly lower than the other, the chiropractor conducted an examination, which also included X-rays. This revealed that Tanner had severe scoliosis (curvature of the spine); which was never mentioned by any other practitioner. Tanner started receiving Chiropractic adjustments with the main focus of reducing vertebral subluxations and restoring nervous system communication.

After only a couple months of Chiropractic care, he began to experience a reduction in the number of seizures during the traditional bad week and a shorter recovery time the following week. His seizure activity was reduced by 50 percent; now experiencing only four to six seizures over the course of the entire bad week. There was also some noticeable improvement in his posture.

Following a few more months of Chiropractic care, there was yet another exciting breakthrough! The cycle, which had been unbreakable for years, was being broken. What emerged could only be explained as stabilizing of seizure activity.

Tanner is not cured of his seizures, but he now only has one or two seizures a month that do not result in the prolonged recovery time that he previously experienced. His speech has improved, becoming quicker and clearer and with less hesitation. His ability to retain and retrieve information is still improving.

The fog is lifting!

Rob Murray, DC
Murray Family Chiropractic
389 Eagle Street
Newmarket, ON L3Y 1K5
905-895-0663
drrob@murraychiropractic.com
www.MurrayChiropractic.com
twitter.com/RobMurrayDC
facebook.com/robmurraydc

Attention Deficit Disorder and More

Dr. Tana K. Frisina

Candace was a pastor's wife and a mother of two boys. She had recently moved to my area and had heard that I worked with children of all ages.

She was curious if Chiropractic could help her youngest son, Jon, who was diagnosed with ADD.

They had tried a few medications to help him with focus, with little to no help. And one of the side effects of the medications was growth stunting. The young boy's father was six feet six inches and his older brother was going to be nearly as tall. Jon was mostly devastated about his short stature. He was an extremely bright kid who loved to play sports.

After a thorough consultation and examination, it was determined that Jon would benefit from Chiropractic care and nutritional supplementation. Shortly after beginning Chiropractic care, Jon was able to concentrate on his schoolwork; it was estimated that he was approximately 50 percent better. Within a few months, he was able to do his work in school and at home without being so easily distracted. And he had also grown for the first time in over a year—and not just a little. He grew three inches!

Once he was in high school, Jon no longer needed the supplements as long has he continued to get periodic Chiropractic checkups and adjustments when necessary. When he graduated from high school, he said to me, "Doc, I was thinking the other day, that I would not have been able to accomplish this without you. Thank you."

My heart melted. This over six-foot-tall young man was ready to start another chapter in his life, healthy and well, with complete confidence. He is now in college, getting nearly all A's and is still playing baseball.

The Power that made the body, can heal the body.

Tana K. Frisina, DC
Frisina Family Wellness Center
1533 S. MacArthur Blvd.
Springfield, IL 62704
217-787-4345
www.frisinafamilychiropractic.com

Autism and Anxiety

Dr. Tye Moe

When eleven-year-old Korben began coming to Whole Family Chiropractic in October 2014, his mom, Chrissie, was not sure he would sit still for even gentle neurological adjustments. "I had tried everything for Korben's autism and anxiety. I was so scared they would not be able to get him to let them adjust him," Chrissie said. "But they did!

"My son's sessions look so different from when he started just a few months ago. It is really amazing how much he has gained since starting with Dr. Tye and Dr. Chelsey," she said. "Not only have Korben's repetitive behaviors and sounds—flapping hands, jumping on one leg, ripping up paper, making loud noises, and constant movements—decreased drastically,

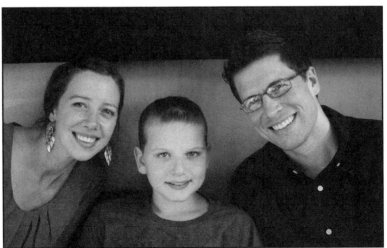

Kids Practice Member of the Month Korben S. with Whole Family Chiropractic's Dr. Chelsey Henney and Dr. Tye Moe

but his anxiety and neediness have significantly decreased too, much to our joy.

"He is able to wait longer and to trust that what he is waiting for will happen. He is able to trust other people more. He is more adventurous. His ability to sit still is far better, and his language is emerging.

"From being completely nonverbal with just signs and a few sounds, he now says about twenty 20 words, and every day he attempts new ones. His language has also become clearer, and he can articulate better," she added. "Before, he would just make a noise."

I also heard good feedback from school on his language, his being more social, and his ability to do work. Korben's mood is better, too. And his accidents have mostly gone away! Before, his parents were dealing with eight to twelve accidents per day, and now they are down to three or less per week!

"It is exciting," Chrissie said. "And, I can tell Korben likes the adjustments at Whole Family Chiropractic. That has not been the case with other therapies!"

Tye Moe, DC
Whole Family Chiropractic
2221 Ford Parkway, Suite 200
St. Paul, MN 55116
651-789-0033
www.healthyfamilymn.com
facebook.com/ChiropractorStPaul

Baby John

Dr. Wendy Coburn

Diagnosed with epilepsy, baby John presented to my office at eleven weeks of age. His mom had a great pregnancy and what she felt a great delivery. John was born at a birthing center with a midwife, no stress, no complications, but very fast.

Within two hours after delivery, baby John had his first adjustment. Shortly after delivery, John was noted to be spitting up a lot and was medicated to control this symptom. He was adjusted by his chiropractor two more times before the family moved to Edmonton, when John was only a couple weeks old.

It was around this time when baby John started having screaming episodes where his arms would extend over his head; these lasted approximately two minutes. These episodes increased in frequency, up to ten to fifteen per day. His mom and dad, obviously concerned, took their child to the local emergency room. Since that time, John has been in and out of hospital, subjected to test after test; MRIs, EEGs, blood work, etc.; all to determine what is wrong.

Medically, the doctors could find nothing wrong, but diagnosed John with epilepsy. There were no tumors or no fractures; no reason for John to be having seizures day after day. Nevertheless, he was prescribed three strong medications to stop the seizures.

Following a three-week stay in hospital, baby John was brought to my office. After a thorough health history and examination, I found stress on his upper neck like I had not seen in a very long time. He also had issues with is tailbone and skull. We adjusted him every day for two weeks. On the day following his third adjustment, Baby John had ten seizures. Since then, he has had only a handful, generally when he is tired.

Progress has continued, and I am now excited to share he has been seizure free for over a week. His personality is starting to shine through and his eyes are glowing. His upper eyelids used to droop and his eyes were cloudy. He is a new boy. Mom is already excited to see how John's health will continue to transform as time goes on.

The power of the human body is absolutely amazing once you remove the interference through Chiropractic.

Wendy Coburn, DC
West Edmonton Family Chiropractic Studio
780-484-2272
www.chiropracticbalance.com

A Renewed Life

Dr. Emir Lervy

T was brought to our office by his parents a few years ago. He was thirteen years old. He arrived in an "adult pushchair" with his head in his lap, completely folded at the hips. This is the way he sat all day long, every day.

At school, they would lay T down so he could see and interact. He made a few sounds and he would grind his teeth constantly. It was obvious that he was very frustrated.

I was told that T had a tumor removed (Medulla Blastoma) when he was three and a half years old. Although it was 98 percent removed, the trauma of the surgery and subsequent chemotherapy left T with retarded mental growth. T was only given a 40 percent chance of survival and the intervention, although successful surgically, did nothing to give him much of a life.

He went from being a happy toddler who was walking and talking, to a young boy who was lying still for most of the day. His parents had little to no hope that T would ever thrive. Of course, they brought him to our office as a last resort. Just maybe, Chiropractic could give T some quality of life—even if just a slight improvement.

After a thorough consultation and examination, it was obvious that T had subluxations and nervous system interference. I had no idea what results might be attained by correcting his subluxations, or whether correction was even possible. I doubted I could help him, but seeing desperation in the eyes of the parents, I thought, *We have nothing to lose.*

In hindsight, I should have trusted innate more than my head! I could have chosen to have faith rather than doubt the human body's ability to adapt and heal.

After only a few weeks of care, to my surprise and everyone else's, T started sitting up straight in his chair. Now, a few years later, he uses a walker to stand up and play, and can even take a few aided steps! He has started to babble again and the teeth grinding is minimal.

When T gets adjusted, he has the most beautiful smile and tries to grab my hand! As interference is removed, the power that made his body is healing his body.

This is obviously not a *full* recovery; however the quality of T's and his family's life has been significantly improved. They have said that he is happier, content, and interacts with his sister and his classmates. He even loves the sensation of wind and rain on his face (which he never did before Chiropractic).

Additionally, T's immunity has improved so enormously he needs less medication. His parents and little sister are having a much more relaxed and fun time with T since he has become more integrated into the family. His sister has noticed so much improvement over the last few years, she now wants T to start walking so he can build a snowman with her at Christmas!

As I keep adjusting him, I remain positive that T can get closer to optimum health—after all, he has to be ready for his formal next year!

Emir Lervy, DC
A Chiropractic Touch
18 Glenmacoffer Road
Omagh, Northern Ireland BT79 7RJ
Emir@lervy.net

Felix's Story

Dr. Joe Kerber

Having a child is one of the most rewarding, and yet sometimes challenging, experiences. As a parent, you want the best for your child. Parents want to make certain their child is happy and healthy. Imagine, though, if your child did not respond to you as you tried to put your love into them; no eye contact or focus, just a lack of engagement from your son.

Three years go by, and the baby you carried for nine months, bonded with, nurtured, and love unconditionally still fails to provide eye contact and focus. He has so many random meltdowns that going out in public is like playing toddler Russian roulette. You want answers, so you take him to medical specialists for help. At the age of three, your son has a diagnosis of autism and a conversation begins to get him on medications.

Fast forward two years and your child is in kindergarten. The teacher states he really struggles with concentration and it interferes with the class. You love your child, so you put him through a nutrition protocol, take him to speech, occupational, and behavioral therapy as last-ditch efforts to avoid drugging him.

Little to no change occurs. The decision to medicate him in the hope that he will have improved concentration is made. You notice little if any change—and you still don't have your son back. Your son is brilliant but struggles through the next five years to socialize and focus, at school and at home.

Your efforts seem futile. Everything you have tried is not working, yet the medical doctor increases the dose of your child's medication. Your frustration and fear continue to rise. You question your parenting skills, you wonder if there is something else you are missing, recognizing your life is a puzzle with a missing piece. With desperation, you get back to researching if there is anything else that has changed in the last seven years since your son's diagnosis was given. Your search reveals that Chiropractic can be beneficial for kids with neurologic issues such as autism and sensory processing.

This is the beginning of the end of Felix's old story.

As a chiropractor, I realize that everyone has a story. Felix's care was intense in frequency; and to say his family was fully committed would be an understatement. After just two weeks of specific Chiropractic care, Felix's mom noticed improvements all around in Felix's life. He began focusing a lot more in school and on small tasks he was asked to perform. His frustration level decreased significantly. He started making eye contact, especially during spontaneous conversation that he never used to participate in. He used to have to be coaxed into doing things, whereas now he was voluntarily jumping to do them.

Felix's mom said, "What you do makes sense, and I see it in my child."

Chiropractic has given her the son she was searching for and knew Felix was. Felix is becoming the boy he was designed to be. For Felix and his family, Chiropractic was the missing piece of the puzzle they looked for more than seven years.

Finally, the puzzle is complete—and looks absolutely exceptional.

Joe Kerber, DC
Strive Chiropractic
3361 45th St., #108
Fargo, ND 58104
701-893-4200
www.strivechiropractic.com
facebook.com/StriveChiropractic

Carlos' Transformation

Dr. Kahlid Mankal

I will always remember the day eight-year-old Carlos was brought into our office by his mother. According to his mom, Carlos did not function well socially or academically and had become very self-loathing. He wanted to die and would often talk about death in general.

This young boy presented with a chief complaint of Attention Deficit Hyperactivity Disorder (ADHD)—inattentive type: anxiety, mood swings, and a learning disability regarding working memory and processing speed.

Seven months prior, private psycho-educational testing had validated these conditions, which permitted several accommodations to be utilized in school, including the following: requesting paraphrasing of instructions to ensure comprehension, allowing extra time to complete assignments, and having printed material read to him.

Regarding behavior issue, Carlos' frustration with his friends and challenges with other students at school caused him considerable anger and frequent outbursts in class. Carlos' mother brought him for Chiropractic care as an alternative treatment plan to manage these concerns. She reported that his medications appeared to be ineffective, causing nausea, heart palpitations and low appetite.

After examining Carlos' posture using thermography and X-ray imaging, we confirmed the presence of vertebral subluxations in his upper neck and sacrum. We also found a major cranial subluxation. We started subluxation-based Chiropractic care and cranial work, which resulted in significant decrease in irritability, temper tantrums, and mood swings; and improved his social interaction, energy, memory, and immune function.

Carlos' mom told us that he has made lots of friends and is smiling and laughing again! After eight months of Chiropractic care, Carlos continues to progress as evidenced by positive reports from his schoolteachers and parents.

I will always remember the powerful words spoken by his mother: "We have our son back!"

Kahlid Mankal, DC
Ottawa, Ontario, Canada
www.barrhavenwellnesscenter.com

Elizabeth's Story

Dr. Katrina Sokolowski

Elizabeth is a beautiful seven-year-old girl who has struggled since she was in her mother's womb. She was delivered at thirty-six weeks via Cesarean section in order to have a shunt placed in her brain. She was born with improper skull formation, which has caused her to live with hydrocephaly.

When I first met Elizabeth, her mother was extremely concerned about Elizabeth's developmental delays. In addition to chronic constipation and bathroom issues, Elizabeth had delays in speech, motor, and sensory planning issues; and apraxia (the inability to perform particular purposeful actions) as a result of brain damage.

Elizabeth has low muscle tone and still wore diapers because one of her delays included the inability to potty train completely. Additionally, her mom was tired of having to give her daughter enemas on a weekly basis. This was described as a difficult task for the entire family. Elizabeth had to be held down in order to receive the enema. Can you imagine the strain on this beautiful little girl and the agony felt by her parents?

Elizabeth began Chiropractic care on a weekly basis to see if we could help. Our first priority was to restore proper nerve function to her body, and hopefully enhance her ability to move her bowels. Within about three weeks, Mom mentioned that Elizabeth had not required an enema to move her bowels in two weeks. What a relief this created for the entire family.

Elizabeth continues with Chiropractic care and has done very well. Since starting care, she has only required one enema; and that was after her shunt had to be replaced. Elizabeth is starting to use the bathroom better and is showing signs of growing. She is also making progress in her balance and motor skills.

Although much of her speech is difficult to understand, she is developing the ability to say some words with greater clarity. Her parents have made Chiropractic a priority in their lives. We will continue to watch Elizabeth improve, grow, and thrive.

Katrina Sokolowski, DC
First Choice Family Chiropractic
2709 Gillionville Rd., Suite 2
Albany, GA 31721
229-594-1546

Erb's Palsy

Dr. Jason Lamarche

My son had what the doctors called a "traumatic birth." Among other things, his left arm had no movement. A couple of months later, after an EMG, the neurologist said my son had Erb's palsy/Shoulder Dystocia, which prevented him from having any movement in his left arm.

My son received therapy through early intervention and also saw a doctor at Shriners Hospital in Oak Park, Illinois. After many medical visits, evaluations, and playing the wait-and-see game for him to build muscle, the doctor thought it was finally time to perform surgery.

When he was three years old, he had a Left Hoffer Transfer, which we understood as basically a transfer of muscle from one part of his arm to the part with the deficit. The surgery went great! He healed well and was able to move his arm higher than ever before.

Although he could raise his arm, he couldn't really turn it. He couldn't button his pants, coat, or anything that required that sort of hand/arm movement. He couldn't wash himself either, or do his hair because he was still very limited in his arm/hand movements.

He started as a patient with Dr. Jason Lamarche at the age of eight. At his first visit, Dr. Lamarche evaluated him. I told Dr. Lamarche what he had been through and my concerns regarding his hand and arm. He looked at my son's elbow and immediately said, "It's locked. His elbow is locked."

I remember feeling mad and skeptical at the same time. Mad, because for eight years no one had ever said anything about his elbow. It was always his muscle and nerves. I was skeptical for the same reason. After all of the medical visits, why had no one ever told us about this issue with his elbow? Was it true and could anything really be done?

Dr. Jason began spinal adjustments and working on my son's elbow and wrist. The moment of skepticism completely disappeared two weeks after my son's first visit when I asked him to move his wrist AND IT MOVED! Although it was slight, it moved. That was the first time in eight years he was able to move his wrist.

Another thing that came as a surprise, only because it had always been a constant, was my son's "wet cough." He had suffered with a constant cough since infancy. It did not seem to be problematic but it was always there. Regardless if the weather was dry, cold, or warm he coughed.

It was earlier this year when I realized I hadn't heard him cough in quite some time. The only thing that had changed in my son's routine was getting Chiropractic care. Although he wasn't being seen or "treated" for his cough, the adjustments put everything in order and his cough was completely gone!

My son is still a Chiropractic client, and it is amazing how much he can do. He can completely bathe himself, which is a big deal for a nine-year-old boy. His left hand is still a work in progress but he can button some pants and tie his own shoes now. I have no doubt he will get there—and wish I would have looked into Chiropractic care sooner.

I've learned many things as I went down this road with my son, and having my son as a patient of Dr. Lamarche has been a truly rewarding learning experience. I never understood how the nervous system fully worked and how important adjustments can be for it to work properly. Now, I do. Thank you, Dr. Lamarche and Chiropractic!

(Submitted by Deb Ritze)

Jason Lamarche, DC
Elite Chiropractic & Rehab
180 E. Main
Braidwood, IL 60408
815-458-2225
elitebraidwood@gmail.com
www.elitechiropracticandrehab.com
facebook.com/drjlamarche

Color My World with Hope

Dr. Monika Buerger

Half of my practice is working with adults who have chronic health issues. The other half is working with children who have chronic health issues and neurodevelopmental challenges, primarily "autism." I purposely use quotation marks around "autism" because I do not like labels. Although some of these children have the signs and symptoms of "autism," so often they are subluxated and toxic and that is what leads to such a label.

Most of the children I work with are severely compromised physiologically as well as developmentally. About half of them are nonverbal; however, they tell me a story with their eyes, their body movements, and their actions.

One little guy told his story through color, and it was a most fabulous story! Thirteen-year-old Ian had a limited vocabulary that was all repetitive in nature. He rarely slept, instead pacing around the house, and had a near constant "stammer" with his hands. He would have severe anger outbursts and had a difficult time sitting still. He also suffered with gastrointestinal issues.

Many "autistic" children do not like to be touched, as they are often hypersensitive to sensory stimulation. Ian was no exception. Unfortunately, this can make it difficult to adjust these children. During our first meeting, it was also clear that Ian was constantly on the move. Essentially, he was a severe hyperactive, hyper-sensory child with a lot of adrenaline pushing through his body. I knew how important it was that I gain his trust prior to trying to adjust him.

Understanding that so much "autistic behavior" stems from gastrointestinal distress, I decided that I would start with trying some visceral manipulation to see how he would respond. We started this work "on the run" as he moved quickly about the room. Soon, his body began to relax and he was able to lie down on the adjustment table. His mother was amazed as he lay still for a half hour with no fuss. If I moved my hands, he would grab them and place them back on his stomach. On his second visit, he swiftly came into the room and lay down on the adjustment table. At that point, I felt that I had already gained enough trust from the first visit to try adjusting him. Not unexpectedly, his atlas, the first cervical bone, was in need of adjusting. He was a bit hesitant, but I knew how important it was to move forward with the adjustment and free his nervous system so he could start to heal.

Fast forward ... every subsequent visit has been Ian reminding his mother of his appointments. I can barely get into the room fast enough for him because he is so eager to get adjusted. He is less repetitive in conversation, sleeps better, experiences less gastrointestinal issues, and in better overall health. However, there is one thing in particular that really

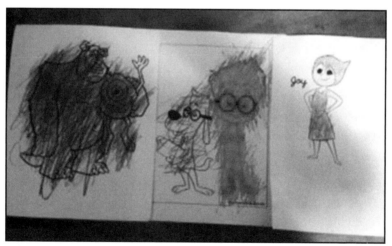

Left: Ian's first picture about one month into care; uses two colors.

Middle: Note the improvement within the lines; uses two colors

Right: About nine months into care; smaller picture and maintains good line integrity. Uses four colors in an appropriate manner.

tells Ian's story. About one month after his first adjustment, his mother came in and, with tears in her eyes, she said, "Ian has started asking to color."

Prior to Chiropractic care, he had no interest in coloring or any other activities. The light was definitely starting to shine in this beautiful, loving, little guy!

Monika Buerger, BA, DC
Eagle Canyon Wellness & Sensory Development Center
1516 S. Midway Ave.
Ammon, ID 83406
208-346-7763

Index of Contributing Doctors